EPIDEMIOLOGY
AND
HEALTH SERVICES

EPIDEMIOLOGY————
AND————————
HEALTH SERVICES————

Haroutune K. Armenian
Sam Shapiro

New York   Oxford
Oxford University Press
1998

Oxford University Press

Oxford   New York
Athens   Auckland   Bangkok   Bogota   Bombay
Buenos Aires   Calcutta   Cape Town   Dar es Salaam
Delhi   Florence   Hong Kong   Istanbul   Karachi
Kuala Lumpur   Madras   Madrid   Melbourne
Mexico City   Nairobi   Paris   Singapore
Taipei   Tokyo   Toronto   Warsaw

and associated companies in
Berlin   Ibadan

Copyright © 1998 by Oxford University Press, Inc.

Published by Oxford University Press, Inc.
198 Madison Avenue, New York 10016

Oxford is a registered trademark of Oxford University Press

Library of Congress Cataloging-in-Publication Data
Armenian, Haroutune K.
Epidemiology and health services /
Haroutune K. Armenian, Sam Shapiro.
p.   cm. Includes bibliographical references and index.
ISBN 0–19–509359–3
1. Epidemiology. 2. Public health—Research.
I. Shapiro, Sam. II. Title.
[DNLM: 1. Epidemiologic Methods—Great Britain.
2. Health Services Research—Great Britain.
WA 950 A728e 1998]
RA652.A76   1998
362.1′072—dc21
DNLM/DLC
for Library of Congress   97–856

1 2 3 4 5 6 7 8 9

Printed in the United States of America
on acid-free paper

PREFACE

In an environment where the growth in health care expenditures must be contained without compromising access to and quality of care, a rational process of decision making is essential. Professionals dealing with problems of health care delivery need to have a grounding in scientific approaches. Although many textbooks and specialized publications have successfully and systematically presented epidemiologic methods to the interested apprentice and scholar, most of these texts have not discussed these methods within the actual context of problem solving in health services.

What is the relevance of epidemiology to the decision-making process within the health services? Can epidemiology help to resolve some of the core issues of health care delivery systems? If we are limited in our ability to launch large-scale interventions and experimental studies, what are some alternative approaches to study design? How can we best make use of routinely collected data from surveillance and other information systems? How can we best synthesize information to make more reasonable inferences? These are some of the questions that *Epidemiology and Health Services* tries to answer. It aims to make epidemiology part of the decision process in health services delivery and to help health care managers understand and appreciate the appropriate use of epidemiologic methods.

This book demonstrates the relevance of epidemiologic methods to health services, describes their strengths and limitations, and offers approaches for making pertinent inferences. Each of the methods is discussed in the context of actual cases or problems.

Part I presents three strategies for the practice of public health, health services research, and program development. These approaches have been selected because they are practical and because they provide a framework for problem investigation and problem solving. These introductory chapters also give the necessary grounding in terminology to help readers progress through the second part of the book. The first chapter presents an overview of the epidemiologic methods commonly used to provide the information base for decisions about health services. The basic approach described in this chapter is that of epidemiologic problem investigation. The second chapter is focused on a six-step approach of problem solving that is used to address important issues in public health. The third chapter describes an approach to program development and evaluation at the intersection of epidemiology and public policy.

Part II applies the most important methods in epidemiology to health services research and development. Each of the nine chapters in this section first presents a theoretical overview of the specific methods under consideration. This is followed by a discussion of case studies based on published studies of health services. A number of questions guide the reader through the most salient issues of these case studies.

This is a book that addresses the needs of a broad spectrum of health professionals. It will help health services administrators, managers, and other professionals design and conduct evaluative and intervention research on the delivery of health services. In addition, epidemiology students seeking a broader perspective on methodologic applications of the discipline should benefit from the text.

Baltimore, MD   Haroutune K. Armenian
March, 1997   Sam Shapiro

CONTENTS

Contributors

Haroutune K. Armenian, M.D., Dr.P.H.
Professor
Department of Epidemiology
School of Hygiene and Public Health
The Johns Hopkins University
Baltimore, Maryland

William W. Eaton, Ph.D.
Professor
Department of Mental Hygiene
School of Hygiene and Public Health
The Johns Hopkins University
Baltimore, Maryland

Steven N. Goodman, M.D., Ph.D.
Associate Professor
Department of Oncology/Biostatistics
Johns Hopkins Medical Institutions
Baltimore, Maryland

Bernard Guyer, M.D.
Professor and Chair
Department of Maternal and Child Health
School of Hygiene and Public Health
The Johns Hopkins University
Baltimore, Maryland

Donald R. Hoover, Ph.D.
Associate Professor
Department of Epidemiology
School of Hygiene and Public Health
The Johns Hopkins University
Baltimore, Maryland

Sam Shapiro, B.S.
Professor Emeritus
Department of Health Policy
    and Management
School of Hygiene and Public Health
The Johns Hopkins University
Baltimore, Maryland

Donald M. Steinwachs, Ph.D.
Professor and Chair
Department of Health Policy
    and Management
School of Hygiene and Public Health
The Johns Hopkins University
Baltimore, Maryland

Donna F. Stroup, Ph.D., M.Sc.
Associate Director for Science
Epidemiology Program Office
Centers for Disease Control and
    Prevention
Atlanta, Georgia

Stephen B. Thacker, M.D., M.Sc.
Director, Epidemiology Program
    Office
Centers for Disease Control and
    Prevention
Atlanta, Georgia

PART I

Framework
for Action

CHAPTER 1

Problem Investigation in Epidemiology

HAROUTUNE K. ARMENIAN

A retired physician calls the State Health Department requesting an investigation in her neighborhood. She has heard of 12 cases of cancer in the vicinity of her residence during a period of 4 years and would like "to get to the root of the problem." (Example 1)

How should the State Health Department handle such a request? Is this even a problem that should be addressed at the state level? What are the methods that will allow an assessment of the relative importance of this problem? How should the problem be delineated and defined?

The Ministry of Health in Mardounia is under strong political pressure to introduce a law requiring compulsory vaccination for cholera using a new vaccine that has been on the market for about a year and is being distributed by a number of government agencies. (Example 2)

What data do the Ministry of Health need to make an appropriate decision? Does the Ministry need to consider information that goes beyond the efficacy of the vaccine? Are there any special studies that need to be done in Mardounia? If the decision is made to start the vaccination program, how will its impact in Mardounia be evaluated?

Routine statistical data collected at Olympus Hospital show higher fatality rates in patients admitted over the past 2 years compared with rates from a similar period a decade ago. (Example 3)

How should any judgment about the significance of these observations be made? How can such an observation be investigated further?

These are three examples of problems that could be addressed using epidemiologic methods. Epidemiologists have developed systematic approaches that help provide answers to many questions facing health professionals. For these professionals at various levels of decision-making, epidemiologists have the tools to generate information and to conduct a systematic process of making inferences. In the first example, of a suspected increase in the number of cancer cases in a neighborhood, when the state epidemiologist decides to look into the request, details about the cases must be reviewed, diagnoses validated, and expectations of numbers of cancer cases within a similar community established for comparison. The state epidemiologist could also study unusual patterns or characteristics in these cases and decide, based on such data as well as other clinical information, whether the concerns of the reporting physician are warranted and further investigations are needed.

This chapter will (1) introduce epidemiology within the context of delivery of health services, (2) present epidemiologic terminology that will be used within the book, (3) discuss a framework of methods commonly used by epidemiologists in a variety of situations, and (4) describe the process of making inferences.

Role of Epidemiology

Epidemiology is an information science. Data generated with epidemiologic methods may be critical for a number of decisions. Epidemiology generates the data for decisions made at the level of the community or the individual practitioner about investigating problems or prescribing appropriate intervention. Table 1-1 lists a number of areas where appropriate decisions may depend on information generated with epidemiologic methods. In Example 2, about deciding on compulsory use of a new vaccine against cholera in Mardounia, the Ministry of Health has to review both laboratory and clinical data about the vaccine, study the results from a number of clinical vaccine trials, and ascertain the short- and long-term side effects. Since the vaccine is already being distributed in the country, the Ministry of Health may also decide to conduct its own case-control study of the vaccine's effectiveness within Mardounia.

Table 1-1. Areas for decisions that need epidemiologic information

Efficacy
Effectiveness
Compliance
Quality assurance
Planning
Programming
Monitoring
Evaluation
Community diagnosis

Thus, in addition to assessing *efficacy,* or establishing whether a particular intervention works in the best of circumstances, epidemiologists also assess *effectiveness,* or establishing that it works in an environment of regular use within the community. Epidemiologists are also involved in assessing factors affecting adherence to prescribed regimens, or *compliance;* quality of medical care; and other problems of evaluation of performance. Data generated by epidemiologic studies are very useful for the planning and development of programs (see Chapter 3).

Epidemiology is a set of methods as well as an approach for judging the significance of observations and data. Epidemiology is also knowledge that is accumulated over the years about the characteristics and determinants of specific diseases or health conditions. Thus, when we refer to the epidemiology of coronary artery disease, the body of knowledge we are dealing with includes the age and sex distributions of this disease as well as risk factors, like cigarette smoking and lack of physical exercise, that act as determinants of the incidence of the condition. Similarly, the epidemiology of primary health care includes patterns of utilization by age and sex as well as economic, organizational, and other cultural determinants of access to, and utilization of, primary health care. In reviewing the patient fatality rates from Olympus Hospital, we need to know the problems with data collection that underlie false estimates of such rates as well as the actual causes of variation in case fatality rates in similar hospitals.

Epidemiologic methods have developed primarily from active public health problem-solving. Whether it is cholera in mid-nineteenth-century London or the rising cost of health care in the United States in recent decades, epidemiology is involved in problem-solving at a variety of levels. The process of identifying solutions to these problems has enriched epidemiologic methodology by integrating within the discipline a number of new investigative techniques. The widening scope of the problems addressed by epidemiologists has enlarged the circle of health professionals who use epidemiologic methods as part of their practice. Thus, in addition to public health departments, epidemiology today is practiced in hospitals by hospital epidemiologists, clinical epidemiologists, and a number of clinicians and researchers. Epidemiology is practiced in health services research and development, planning, quality assurance, evaluative research, primary health care, and any situation that involves the systematic scrutiny of a health problem and the development of appropriate solutions (Donabedian, 1990; Hulka, 1978; Shapiro, 1991).

Such a systematic approach to problem investigation has led epidemiologists to develop paradigms that have organized investigative strategies. The current paradigm for problem investigation used by epidemiologists has evolved from models established earlier in this century in the acute problem-solving situation of outbreak investigation. Table 1-2 provides a list of the typical steps in outbreak

Table 1-2. Steps in epidemic investigation

1. Define the problem. Is it an epidemic? What is the etiologic agent?
2. Appraise existing data. Determine the date and hour of onset; make an epidemic curve. Prepare a spot map of cases; consider home, work, and places of recreation and special meetings. Where did exposure occur? Calculate attack rates if possible.
3. Formulate a hypothesis.
4. Test the hypothesis. Search for added cases; evaluate all of the data; perform laboratory investigations.
5. Draw conclusions and devise practical applications. Write a report. Undertake long-term surveillance and prevention.

Source: Evans (1982a,b).

investigation. The key steps are ascertaining the validity of the problem, then developing and testing a hypothesis, which includes the important phases of applying judgment to the data that have been collected and of communicating the appropriate information to the public or the decision-makers.

Problem Investigation

As stated previously, the epidemiologic investigation of a health problem involves a number of steps for collecting the appropriate information and for making appropriate inferences. Tables 1-3 and 1-4 list the steps discussed in this section.

Table 1-3. The information-gathering process

1. Ascertain the problem.
2. Review the literature.
3. Use descriptive epidemiology (available data).
      For the problem under study, review:
          Chronology/history (time)
          Geographic distribution (place)
          Demographic characteristics (persons)
      Use indicators of:
          Mortality
          Morbidity (incidence, prevalence)
          Disability, dissatisfaction, etc.
      Generate a hypothesis.
4. Test the hypothesis using analytic designs:
      Cross-sectional
      Case-control
      Cohort
5. Design experiments in animals or humans (if appropriate).

Table 1-4. Process of inferences

1. Assess the existence of *bias* or *artifacts;* review the *validity* or *reliability* of the data.
2. Review possible alternative explanations due to *confounding* through *indirect associations.*
3. Evaluate the association as to causal significance using the *criteria for judgment:*
   Time sequence
   Strength
   Specificity
   Dose response
   Coherence
   Consistency
4. Provide an appropriate explanation for the association. Look for interactions with other variables of interest.

In the first stage of an investigation, we need to ascertain the existence, the magnitude, and the public health significance of the problem. We also need to review the accumulated knowledge about this problem from published material. The data and the tools used to obtain the information for an assessment of the problem are often specific to the situation and the problem under consideration. Five deaths in 1 month of young patients admitted to a hospital for elective surgery call for immediate action. Few professionals would question the need to investigate such a problem. However, five deaths in the same hospital of 85-year-old patients over a whole year may not prompt any thought of an investigation. In the first example, we first need to ascertain the validity of the information—for example, by reviewing the records of these five patients. At this stage, we also need to identify other cases, if any, that have been missed by the initial reports, to trace the magnitude of the problem. A review of the literature about known causes of unexpected deaths in hospitalized children may help develop hypotheses about the etiology of the cases under investigation. The literature may also reveal methods that have been used previously in investigating similar problems.

The second stage of the epidemiologic investigation of a health problem is to determine the parameters of distribution of the problem and to characterize the subgroups affected by it. This is the stage of descriptive epidemiology. Information used for this step is based on data that are usually available from previously collated statistical material or from the initial review of the cases under investigation. Thus, if the problem under investigation is the cost of medical care in community hospitals in Sylvania, we need to review the statistical data about cost from these hospitals. In reviewing such statistical data, epidemiologists systematically pose three questions to determine the dimensions of the problem and to help develop hypotheses that may explain its cause(s): *When? Where?* and *Who?* Answers to these questions will inform us about the historic, geographic, and demographic dimensions of the problem. For any unusual patterns identified through these inquiries, we may be able to develop pertinent hypotheses about the etiology and determinants of the problem.

A review of the time trends of the cost of medical care in Sylvania will help us distinguish whether increases in such costs have been, for example, gradual or sudden. If the changes are sudden, we may be able to identify some changes in the system of care or in accounting and cost mechanisms that have been introduced over a short period of time. In this study of the time dimension, we may also be interested in the seasonal variation of the occurrence of the problem. Such variation may be caused by seasonal patterns of behavior or system modification.

The geographic distribution of the problem will help us delineate better what is of prime interest for us. Are the increases in cost of care similar across all administrative and political units in Sylvania? Are there any unusual foci of extremely high or extremely low costs? What are the characteristics of these extremes?

Similarly, a number of questions help us to understand the demographic distribution of the problem under investigation. Does the high cost of medical care involve to a larger extent older patients or female patients? Are all economic and occupational groups involved similarly with the high cost of medical care in Sylvania?

Based on a review of the data generated in response to these inquiries, a number of hypotheses forming the basis for the analytic investigations that will follow this second stage of our problem investigation can be developed. If the change in cost of medical care in Sylvania is limited to older female patients who are hospitalized during the first 6 months of the year, then we may begin considering a hypothesis of bias due to various issues of measurement or an explanation based on potential confounding by an alternative factor. It is important to note here that, in a number of situations where such descriptive data may be sufficient for our decisions or when our available resources do not allow us to conduct any further special studies that involve new data generation, this is the stage at which our problem investigation may terminate.

The third stage of our investigation involves testing the hypotheses that have been generated. This is the stage of analytic epidemiology, where we use special observational and experimental methods that generate new data. In a study that aims at establishing a relation between an agent and its outcome, it is most important to determine the antecedence of exposure to the agent prior to the development of the outcome. Thus, analytic study designs aim at establishing such a time sequence between exposure and development of the outcome.

We may choose a cohort design, whereby we can identify the study population by exposure patterns and determine the rates of outcome in various exposure groups. Such a design is a direct test of the hypothesis under consideration. Hempelman et al. (1975) suspected that therapeutic exposure to x-rays for enlargement of the thymus in children caused neoplasms of the thyroid. They conducted a cohort study by identifying a group of children who had received such x-ray treatment and compared the incidence of thyroid neoplasms in this group with the incidence of these neoplasms in their siblings who were not exposed to therapeutic x-rays as children. Children exposed to x-rays had over a 20-fold increase in thyroid tumors compared with their nonexposed siblings during two decades of follow-up.

The other major type of observational epidemiologic design is the case-control method. This is the prime example of case-based designs that has been increasingly applied over the past four decades. In this design, the study groups are identified by the presence or absence of the outcome, and these groups are compared as to the frequency of the exposure in the time period prior to the development of the outcome. (Chapter 8 presents in detail the case-control method as an epidemiologic problem-solving tool.) To determine whether the presence of latrines at home was protective against diarrheal disease in Lesothan children, Daniels et al. (1990) identified cases of diarrhea from primary care facilities and compared the frequency of the presence of latrines in the homes of these children with the same frequency in a control group of children with no diarrhea selected from the same primary care facilities. Using the case-control method, they were able to estimate that children with latrines at home may experience 24% fewer episodes of diarrhea than children from households without a latrine in this population.

In addition to these observational methods where the investigator does not interfere in the natural course of events, epidemiologists and health services researchers use experimental methods. The details of the experimental design and the randomized trial are presented in Chapter 9. The investigator randomly allocates volunteers to experimental and control groups. The experimental group receives the intervention under investigation, and the control group is spared such exposure. As in the cohort study, the groups of exposure are compared as to the incidence of the outcome of interest. One of the simplest randomized trials is the test of efficacy of a new vaccine. A population of volunteer participants is allocated at random to receive the new vaccine or a placebo. The first outcome of interest is the incidence of the side effects of the new vaccine. The incidence of the side effects in the experimental group receiving the new vaccine is compared with the incidence of side effects in the control group. Similarly, to demonstrate efficacy, the incidence of the disease that the vaccine is supposed to protect against is compared in the experimental and control groups.

Inferences

As listed in Table 1-4, whenever data are scrutinized by epidemiologists, there is a process of inferences that must be used to arrive at rational conclusions. At each step in the generation of epidemiologic data, we need to assess the validity of the data, the possibility that an alternative factor(s) may underlie and explain the observed association between an outcome and the hypothesized etiology, and the significance of the finding under consideration.

The mandatory first step of this process is to rule out the possibility that the observations under consideration are the result of bias or systematic error. For example, could the higher fatality rates observed at the Olympus Hospital over the past 2 years be due to changes in the classification of deaths within this hospital or to some other artifactual change in the way deaths are enumerated? How does the possibility of such a systematic error affect our ability to make appropriate inferences about the reasons for higher fatality rates in this hospital?

Epidemiologists face a number of biases in any investigation. It is important to be aware of the various errors and to handle them at either the design or the analysis phase of the study. We may not be able to eliminate all systematic measurement errors, but it is important to try to measure or estimate the effect that particular biases may have on the results of the study. Within Olympus Hospital, we may be able to review all of the changes that have occurred in the recording and analysis of deaths as well as the measurement of denominators for the various rates used over the years. If such changes and errors are identified, it is important to estimate the size of the effect such an error may have on the results. If the recent change in the classification of deaths gives us a 10% systematic increase in the number of deaths in recent years, could such a change explain a 50% increase in case fatality rates in this hospital?

Following ascertainment of possible biases, the next step in the process of inferences is to look for *confounders,* or other variables that may explain the relation. Epidemiologists deal with confounders at either the design or the analysis phase of the study. In the study by Hempelman et al. (1975), it may be that the higher incidence of thyroid neoplasms in the group exposed to therapeutic x-rays is due to the original thymic enlargement of the exposed group rather than to x-ray exposure in childhood. Thus, thymic enlargement could be the confounder in this observed association between x-rays in childhood and thyroid neoplasms. However, such was not the case since a number of the nonexposed children had thymic enlargement and no increase in risk for thyroid neoplasms. Details of the various methods of dealing with confounders are discussed in Chapter 11.

To assess the significance of a finding, in the next phase of the inferential process, a number of criteria need to be fulfilled if the relation is to be accepted as direct or causal. As stated previously, establishing the time sequence between the agent and the outcome is the most critical of these criteria. Consistency of the finding with similar observations; its strength, as measured by the size of the

Table 1-5. Epidemiologic methods and inferences matrix

		Inferences		
		Assess for Bias	Review for Confounding	Provide a Causal Model
Methods	Descriptive *Mortality* *Morbidity*			
	Analytic *Surveys* *Case-control* *Cohort*			
	Experimental			

relative risk or its estimate; its biologic plausibility, or coherence with the known facts about the phenomenon under study; and the type of relation of the factor and outcome under study, such as specificity and dose response, are some of the other criteria used for judgment. Further details on approaches in the process of inferences are discussed in Chapter 12.

Table 1-5 summarizes the problem investigation paradigm in epidemiology. The rows in this matrix represent the various tools and methods used in epidemiology to generate the data within the process of problem investigation. The columns represent the process of inferences in epidemiology. The essential message of this matrix is that, at every step of the information-gathering process, we need to address issues of bias or measurement error, potential problems with confounders, and the need to make a judgment about the significance of the finding or observation. Whether we are assessing simple mortality statistics or analyzing data from a complex multicenter controlled clinical trial, the same steps apply with regard to making the appropriate inferences.

Common Threads in Methods of Investigation

The various chapters in this book present investigative techniques that are relevant to problem-solving in the health services. The following steps are important to follow when evaluating or designing epidemiologic investigations in general.

1. *Assessing the existence of the problem.* As stated in the earlier example of outbreak investigation, we want to know whether there is a real problem at hand. The definition of the problem influences the whole approach to the investigation and determines the subgroup of the population to be investigated. Delineation of the problem also affects the scope of generalization that can be made from our findings.

2. *Determining the parameters of the distribution of the problem.* A systematic approach to determining the historic/chronologic, geographic, and demographic parameters of the problem is very valuable in the development of hypotheses. Such a descriptive epidemiologic approach also will allow us to identify the group at risk for the problem.

3. *Selecting the appropriate study design for testing the hypotheses.* This selection is based on the strengths and weaknesses of the various methods, the available resources, and the data at hand.

4. *Using the proper methods of analysis.* A well-designed study may fail if the appropriate analytic methods are not used. Some of these methods are discussed in Chapter 11.

5. *Making reasonable inferences from the results of the analysis and other available information.* The following chapters address this issue from various methodologic perspectives.

This chapter has highlighted a number of uses of epidemiology within the framework of health services research and development. Other examples of such uses of epidemiologic methods are developed throughout this book. The second part of this chapter has presented an overview of epidemiologic methods within the context of a paradigm of problem investigation. The two chapters that follow present in more detail some other paradigms used by practitioners of public health and health services research that are relevant to the discussion for the rest of this book.

References

Daniels, D. L., S. N. Cousens, L. N. Makoae, and R. G Feachem. 1990. A case-control study of the impact of improved sanitation on diarrhea morbidity in Lesotho. *Bull. World Health Organ.,* 68:455–463.

Donabedian, A. 1990. Contributions of epidemiology to quality assessment and monitoring. *Infect. Control Hosp Epidemiol.,* 11:117–121.

Evans, A. S. 1982a. Epidemiological concepts. In: *Viral Infections of Humans. Epidemiology and Control,* edited by A. S. Evans. New York: Plenum Press, pp. 1–7.

Evans, A. S. 1982b. Epidemiological concepts and methods. In: *Bacterial Infections of Humans. Epidemiology and Control,* edited by A. S. Evans and H. A. Feldman. New York: Plenum Press, pp. 8–10.

Hempelman, L. H., W. J. Hall, M. Phillips, et al. 1975. Neoplasms in persons treated with x-rays in infancy: fourth survey in 20 years. *J Nat Cancer Inst.* 55:519–530.

Hulka, B. S. 1978. Epidemiological applications to health services research. *J Community Health,* 4:140–149.

Shapiro, S. 1991. Epidemiology and public policy. *Am J Epidemiol.,* 134:1057–1061.

CHAPTER 2

Problem-Solving in Public Health

BERNARD GUYER

Solving problems in public health is fundamentally different from medical diagnosis and treatment. The difference can be illustrated with the following example. A clinician who treats a hypertensive patient might be quite discouraged with a fall in mean diastolic blood pressure of only 5% over a period of a year of treatment; the individual patient might still be symptomatic and at risk of complications. But an epidemiologist who monitors the blood pressure patterns of a population following the initiation of a community-based intervention program and observes a 5% drop in its mean diastolic blood pressure after 1 year of implementation might be ecstatic because a shift in the population indicator of this magnitude would move a large number of individuals into the normotensive range. The change would then be measured by comparing the distribution of blood pressures before and after the intervention.

Public health professionals (e.g., physicians and nurses) are often educated within a clinical/biomedical framework that gives them an individual patient-based, biomedical orientation to health problems but not a broad orientation to the determinants of health, including socioeconomic status, health services structures and organization, or politics. Since public health is the field that links the biologic basis of health and disease with the social and political processes of society, these public health professionals need broader, more effective problem-solving tools and an epidemiologic orientation to the health of populations.

In this chapter, we develop a set of concepts for addressing public health problems. This public health problem-solving paradigm is more general and comprehensive than many of the other methods used in public health, for example, the epidemiologic problem investigation paradigm described in Chapter 1. Problem-solving includes the following steps:

1. Defining the problem
2. Measuring the magnitude of the problem
3. Developing a conceptual framework for the key determinants of the prob-

lem, including the biologic, epidemiologic, sociocultural, economic, and political determinants
4. Identifying and developing intervention and prevention strategies
5. Setting priorities among strategies and recommending policies
6. Implementing programs and evaluating them

The Problem-Solving Paradigm

The problem-solving paradigm described here is well known to public health practitioners and is frequently used in public health agencies, with modifications to fit particular circumstances. Unfortunately, neither this nor other approaches to public health problem-solving have been well described in the literature. Therefore, in this chapter, each of the key elements of the paradigm is discussed with illustrative examples drawn from two well-known public health problems: (1) the health consequences of tobacco and (2) the failure to achieve adequate levels of childhood immunization.

Problem definition

Defining the problem may be the single most important step in public health problem-solving. It is essential that public health professionals recognize the complexity of defining a problem and how the nature of the definition can affect all other aspects of problem measurement, program development, policy-making, and evaluation.

The importance of problem definition can be demonstrated in the case of tobacco and health. In the early 1950s, research identified cigarette smoking as the cause of a single pathologic condition, lung cancer (Doll and Hill, 1950; Wynder and Graham, 1950; Levin et al., 1950). Such a narrow formulation of the problem leads to a narrow range of program approaches, i.e., smoking cessation among smokers, primarily adults. Progress in research, however, expanded and enlarged the definition of the tobacco problem (U.S. Department of Health and Human Services, 1989). Smoking cigarettes was linked subsequently to cardio-vascular diseases in men and women. Smoking during pregnancy was found to have effects on fetal growth and development (Floyd et al., 1993). The findings of adverse effects of exposure to second-hand smoke broadened the population of concern to nonsmokers, including young children exposed at home and workers in the workplace (U.S. Department of Health and Human Services, 1986; Eriksen et al., 1988; Environmental Protection Agency, 1992). Finally, as evidence became available that tobacco has broad toxic effects (McGinnis and Foege, 1993) and that nicotine is an addictive substance (U.S. Department of Health and Human Services, 1988), the public policy problem was expanded to encompass all aspects of the tobacco industry, including marketing, agriculture, and manufacturing (Bartecchi et al., 1994). The chronologic progress of this changing definition is presented in Table 2-1.

In the case of childhood immunization, the public health problem can be defined, broadly, as the failure to protect young children from communicable diseases by a variety of available vaccines. However, embedded in this broad definition of the problem are a number of competing concepts. For example, one way to define the problem is in terms of disease morbidity and mortality; thus, it does not matter what levels of immunization are achieved in a population or under what circumstances as long as the levels are sufficient to prevent transmission of disease. Policies based on this definition lead to communicable disease control approaches. A second way to define the problem is in terms of immunization coverage in the population; thus, the fact that only about 67% of 2-year-old children are immunized with all of the currently recommended vaccines is a problem even if epidemics are not occurring (Centers for Disease Control, 1994). Policies based on this definition would lead to efforts to improve vaccine coverage levels. A third way to define the problem would be to view immunization coverage levels in children as a manifestation of inadequate access to primary health care services (Guyer and Hughart, 1994). Policies based on this definition would ignore immunization as an isolated service, focus on im-

Table 2-1. Chronology of the health consequences of tobacco

1950	Smoking linked to lung cancer
1960s	Dose-response for smoking and cardiovascular disease
	Smoking linked to emphysema and respiratory disease
1964	First U.S. Surgeon General's report on smoking and health
1970s	Maternal smoking linked to low birth weight and other adverse pregnancy outcomes
1980s	Lung cancer deaths in women surpass breast cancer deaths
	Smoking, oral contraceptives, and cardiovascular disease linked in women
1986	Surgeon General's report linked passive smoking to lung cancer
	Passive maternal smoking linked to childhood asthma
	Passive smoking effects in the workplace
1988	Surgeon General's report linked nicotine and addiction
1990	418,000 deaths attributed to tobacco, including:
	180,000 cardiovascular disease
	120,000 lung cancer
	33,000 other cancers
	85,000 respiratory diseases
	Passive smoking linked to cardiovascular disease
1992	Environmental Protection Agency report: environmental smoking hazard; tobacco smoke as group "A" carcinogen
1994	Food and Drug Administration: nicotine and addiction

proving access to health care, and expect the immunization coverage levels to improve.

Inherent in the consideration of problem definition is the issue of ''who'' sets the definitions and ''how'' definitions are set in our society. Since problem definition has broad implications for magnitude, cost, and consequences, the process is highly political. Problem definitions do not simply come from textbooks. They are arrived at through complex processes involving negotiations among experts, professional panels, interest groups, communities, and legislative and administrative bodies. Certain stakeholders would have the definitions set at their narrowest dimensions; others would create broad definitions. Often, scientific panels are asked to provide their best assessment of the scientific data to arrive at a definition. Even these processes may be altered, however, by administrative agencies, legislative bodies, or the courts through litigation.

Measurement

Problem definition has enormous implications for problem measurement. Measuring the magnitude of a public health problem may begin with the application of measures of incidence and prevalence. The process, however, goes well beyond these descriptive epidemiologic parameters. The measurement process must define the populations at risk, and the nature of those populations has implications for the attention given to problems by society. For example, the British physician study of smoking recognized physicians' risk of cancer related to tobacco (Doll et al., 1994).

Measurement also requires the adoption of indicators that correspond to the problem definition. In the case of childhood immunization, for example, several indicators are available, including those of specific disease morbidity and mortality, overall vaccination coverage, specific vaccine coverage, access to vaccination services, and the quality of primary health care delivery. Specifically, the immunization status of a population of children may be measured by one of four possible measures: (1) up-to-date by 2 years of age, a frequently used indicator and the measure used in the National Objectives for the Year 2000 (U.S. Department of Health and Human Services, 1991a); (2) up-to-date by school entry; (3) age-appropriate immunization, a measure of the closeness with which actual immunizations conform to the recommended age schedules; and (4) immunization status, defined by the incidence of an important vaccine-preventable disease like measles. Table 2-2 indicates the advantages and disadvantages of these various measures.

The case of childhood immunizations provides some important insights into

Table 2-2. Advantages and disadvantages of different indicators of children's immunization status

Indicator[a]	Advantages	Disadvantages
UTD by 2	Well established national objectives Allows for catch-up	Allows for delays
AA immunization	Very precise measure against recommendation	Too precise (trivial delay gets recorded as failure) Need accurate dates
UTD by school age	Easily available Very accurate	Measures problem at too old an age to result in effective policies to protect young children
Measles cases	Important disease	May not reflect low coverage

[a]UTD by 2, up-to-date by 2 years of age; AA immunization, age-appropriate immunization; UTD by school age, up-to-date by school entry.

the complexities of problem measurement and its link to problem definition. It is estimated from surveys of U.S. children entering schools in the first grade (at age 6 years) that more than 99% of these children are fully immunized, leading to the possible conclusion that there is no problem of childhood immunization (Centers for Disease Control, 1991a). Unfortunately, the measles epidemics of 1989 and 1990 showed this not to be the case (Centers for Disease Control, 1989, 1990, 1991a, b). Retrospective surveys in cities with epidemics showed that only 11–60% of 2-year-old children were fully immunized (Centers for Disease Control, 1992). Thus, the school-based data were misleading because they assessed the wrong indicator in the wrong population. In fact, the best measure of the risk of vaccine-preventable diseases to U.S. children might come from assessments of coverage in children in the poorest sections of U.S. cities in the first year of life because these levels are predictive of receipt of additional vaccinations. Despite recent national efforts to raise coverage levels, these populations may still be at risk.

Key determinants and conceptual frameworks

Mosley and Chen (1984) developed a key-determinants framework for examining the array of proximal and distal factors that relate to the premature death of young children in developing countries. Theirs is an excellent example of a conceptual framework for organizing the complex set of biologic risk factors, demographic and socioeconomic variables, and environmental considerations that must be understood in order to address important public health problems. Rarely do these problems have a simple "cause."

The purpose of conceptual frameworks is to organize disparate risk factors into a set of domains that are linked in a logical fashion to the outcome and can become the organizing principle for intervention strategies. In the case of tobacco and its health consequences, the domains that influence the problem include the following: the initiation and development of personal behaviors with deleterious health consequences, the widespread marketing of tobacco products, the addictive effects of nicotine, environmental exposure to second-hand smoke, and the agricultural and economic place of tobacco in a worldwide economy.

In the case of low childhood immunization status, three domains influence whether children receive appropriate immunizations (Cutts et al., 1992): the behavior of their parents in seeking preventive health care, including their knowledge and attitudes; the barriers to access to that care, including the cost of vaccines, insurance coverage for preventive health care, availability of services, demographic characteristics, and a societal commitment to immunization in the form of public health policies; and the ability of health care providers to effectively deliver immunizations, including the likelihood that "missed opportunities" for immunization will occur. The conceptual framework shown in Figure 2-1 relates these domains to immunization outcome.

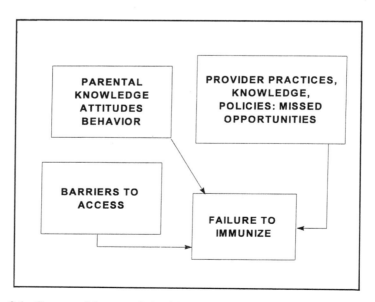

Figure 2-1. Conceptual framework for failure to immunize children.

Strategies for intervention and prevention

Prevention programs must use a conceptual framework to develop a full array of interventions and to be fully informed in choosing the most effective policy. Without a complete set of intervention alternatives, public policy may jump at expedient programs that prove in the long run to be ineffective and discredited. Strategic thinking requires a complete set of alternatives from which to make decisions.

One of the best public health tools for such strategy development comes from the field of injury control: the Haddon matrix. This systematic framework for injury prevention organizes potential strategies into a 3×3 table with "host," "agent," and "environment" factors along one dimension and "preevent," "event," and "postevent" time periods along the other dimension (National Committee for Injury Prevention and Control, 1989). The cells of the matrix can then be used to develop the full range of potential interventions at any stage of an injury event.

In relation to the problem of tobacco, the National Cancer Institute has developed a conceptual framework for the sequence of steps that characterize the progression from the nonsmoking adolescent to the dependent adult smoker (Figure 2-2) (U.S. Department of Health and Human Services, 1991b). The framework lays out a logical sequence and then identifies the factors that encourage the progress from one stage to the next (on the left side of the figure) and the countermeasures that would prevent this progression (on the right side of the figure). This framework supports the importance of a systematic logical approach.

Setting priorities and policy formulation

Public health professionals may take responsibility for much of the problem-solving process to this point in the paradigm, but they must understand that policy-making is a complex political process that goes well beyond professional expertise alone. To be effective in this policy arena, health professionals must understand the positions of all of the stakeholders in any policy decision. Failure to recognize the realities and opportunities of policy- making will result in disillusionment, frustration, and incompetence.

First, the policy-making process can be thought of as involving three elements: a *knowledge base, political will,* and *social strategies.* The *knowledge base* refers to all of the information needed to make a policy decision. Public health professionals play an important part in bringing this knowledge to the attention of policymakers. The knowledge base contains much of the information already described, including the definition of the problem and quantitative estimates of its magnitude. The knowledge base should also include information

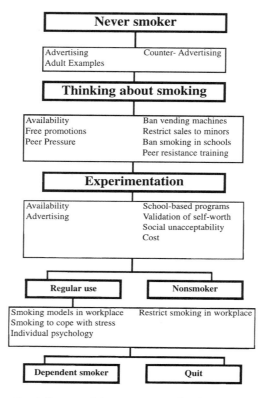

Figure 2-2. Forces that influence adolescent progression into adult smoking.

about the cost and consequences of the problem and evaluate information about the variety of programmatic solutions and their likelihood of success. *Political will* refers to the willingness of policymakers, who are most often elected officials in either the legislative or executive branches of government, to tackle a particular problem and reach a policy direction. Finally, *social strategies* are those broad themes used by society to solve problems. In public health, for example, these strategies may include the development of laws and regulations to govern or restrict certain behaviors; the development of a variety of direct service programs; the provision of governmental funds through grants, contracts, or individual entitlements; or the reliance on marketplace economic forces to encourage particular policy directions.

Second, public health professionals must understand the roles and positions of the various stakeholders in the policy decision. In relation to policy concerning tobacco and health, the stakeholders are well known and hold powerful positions.

Among these is the tobacco industry, which has resisted any intrusion from governmental public health or regulatory agencies into its business, even to the point of denying the accepted causal relation between tobacco and adverse health outcomes. The tobacco industry also represents, often, a wide variety of stakeholders who profit from societal consumption of tobacco; these include farmers, marketers, advertisers, bar and restaurant owners, other merchants, the media, and, ironically, governments that receive tax revenue from tobacco sales. Economic self-interest defines these interest groups. They become crucially involved in the public health debate over controlling tobacco. Public interest groups and advocacy organizations are also stakeholders and will attempt to influence a process. Groups representing the families of victims who have suffered the consequences are important. Professional organizations, health care providers, and health care institutions have become active around these issues. Finally, the public health agencies themselves need to be viewed as stakeholders in this complex political process.

Third, the policy-making process involves the selection of policy directions among alternative strategies. To the extent that policymakers have considered the full range of strategies and have weighed all of the consequences of each, they are capable of making an informed decision. Public health professionals can play a critical role in fully informing policymakers of this aspect during the process. In the case of childhood immunization, for example, three broad alternative strategies evolve from the conceptual framework described earlier. Table 2-3 indicates how policy directions will follow from the formulation of the nature of the problem and from the possible intervention strategies. By having all of this information, policymakers can choose effective approaches. The failure to develop a complete and fully informed set of policy alternatives may result in ineffective policy development.

Table 2-3. Policy alternatives to improve immunization coverage among young children

Strategic Intervention	Policy Alternatives
Change parental behavior	Educate parents
	Penalize welfare recipients who miss visits for their children's immunizations
Remove barriers to access	Require insurance coverage for vaccines
	Mobile vans to deliver immunizations to homes
	Government to purchase and distribute all vaccines
Improve provider practices	Educate providers about missed opportunities
	Develop registries and tracking systems
	Feedback to providers on their coverage levels

Implementation and evaluation

Implementation is the process by which policy decisions are translated into programmatic activity. *Evaluation* is the process of measuring the success with which programs reach their stated objectives. These two processes are integrally related and essential elements of public health problem-solving.

Implementation begins when the legislative branch of government passes legislation and hands a mandate over to the executive branch for implementation. *Program implementation* is a set of administrative activities that translate the legislative intent into programmatic reality. Key steps in this implementation process include the following: effective communication concerning all aspects of the program to all levels of personnel involved in program delivery; development of procedures and administrative mechanisms that ensure program effectiveness; allocation of financial and other resources at levels adequate to meet expectations; and development of monitoring and data systems needed to measure program progress, to support accountability, and to evaluate effectiveness. Chapters 3 and 4 expand on these areas. Policy implementation, program development, and evaluation are carried out primarily by public health professionals working in agencies.

In the case of childhood immunization, the importance of program implementation and evaluation can be demonstrated with case material from a measles outbreak that occurred in Milwaukee, Wisconsin, in 1989 (Schlenker and Fessler, 1990). In that state, all Medicaid children were enrolled in managed care organizations (health maintenance organizations) so that each child had a designated provider. Further, these providers were paid a ''capitated'' fee per month, in advance, to provide all necessary preventive and curative care to the children enrolled in their organization. Despite this arrangement, which sounded ideal for ensuring adequate access to primary care, the investigation of the measles epidemic found that the highest attack rates occurred among Medicaid children enrolled in these managed care organizations. In fact, these providers were collecting their capitation payments for the children but not ensuring that the immunization services were actually being provided. Thus, while the program was developed on sound policy, it failed to implement that policy and to evaluate its impact. The epidemic of measles became the first indicator of a problem.

Conclusion

The Institute of Medicine report *The Future of Public Health* (Committee for the Study of the Future of Public Health, 1988) concluded that the field of public health was in ''disarray,'' in part, because public health agencies were no longer clear about their mission and functions. These doubts about the role of public health were echoed during the health care reform debate of 1994. Much of this confusion over the role of public health derives from the failure to understand health problems on the populational level and to address health concerns with methods that link their biologic, epidemiologic, sociologic, political, and economic aspects. In this chapter, we have presented a public health problem-solving paradigm that attempts to achieve these objectives. There is no claim made that this paradigm is unique or exclusive. Public health students and professionals are encouraged to adapt these ideas to their own particular situations and to modify the approach to meet their own needs and experience. The goal of this chapter is to give public health professionals a place to start in the development of their own ideas about making public health policy more effective in improving the public's health.

References

Bartecchi, C. E., T. D. MacKenzie, and R. W. Schrier. 1994. The human costs of tobacco use. *N. Engl. J. Med.*, 330:907–912, 975–980.

Centers for Disease Control. 1989. Measles—United States, first 26 weeks. *Morb. Mortal. Wkly. Rep.*, 38:863–866, 871–872.

Centers for Disease Control. 1991a. Measles vaccination levels among selected groups of preschool-aged children—United States. *Morb. Mortal. Wkly. Rep.*, 40:36–39.

Centers for Disease Control. 1991b. Measles—United States, 1990. *Morb. Mortal. Wkly. Rep.*, 40:369–372.

Centers for Disease Control and Prevention. 1992. Retrospective assessment of vaccination coverage among school-aged children—selected U.S. cities, 1991. *Morb. Mortal. Wkly. Rep.*, 41:103–107.

Centers for Disease Control and Prevention. 1994. Vaccination coverage of 2-year-old children—United States. 1993. *Morb. Mortal. Wkly. Rep.*, 43:705–709.

Committee for the Study of the Future of Public Health, U.S. Institute of Medicine. 1988. *The Future of Public Health.* Washington, D.C.: National Academy Press.

Cutts, F. T., W. A. Orenstein, and R. H. Bernier. 1992. Causes of low preschool immunization coverage in the United States. *Annu. Rev. Public Health*, 13:385–398.

Doll, R., and A. B. Hill. 1950. Smoking and carcinoma of the lung: preliminary report. *BMJ*, 1:739–748.

Doll, R., R. Peto, K. Wheatley, et al. 1994. Mortality in relation to smoking: 40 years' observations on male British doctors. *BMJ*, 309:901–911.

Environmental Protection Agency. 1992. *Respiratory Effects of Passive Smoking: Lung Cancer and Other Disorders.* Washington, D.C.: Office of Health and Environmental Assessment.

Eriksen, M. P., C. A. LeMaistre, and G. R. Newell. 1988. Health hazards of passive smoking. *Annu. Rev. Public Health*, 9:47–70.

Floyd, R. L., B. K. Rimer, G. A. Giovino, et al. 1993. A review of smoking in pregnancy: effects on pregnancy outcomes and cessation efforts. *Annu. Rev. Public Health*, 14:379–411.

Guyer, B., and N. Hughart. 1994. Increasing childhood immunization coverage by improving the effectiveness of primary health care systems for children. *Arch. Pediatr. Adolesc. Med.,* 148:901–902.

Levin, M. L., H. Goldstein, and P. R. Gerhardt. 1950. Cancer and tobacco smoking; a preliminary report. *JAMA,* 143:336–338.

McGinnis, J. M., and W. H. Foege. 1993. Actual causes of death in the United States. *JAMA,* 270:2207–2212.

Mosley, W. H., and L. C. Chen. 1984. An analytical framework for the study of child survival in developing countries. In: *Child Survival; Strategies for Research. A Supplement to Population and Development Review,* vol. 10, edited by W. H. Mosley and L. C. Chen. New York: The Population Council.

National Committee for Injury Prevention and Control. 1989. *Injury Prevention: Meeting the Challenge.* New York: Oxford University Press.

Schlenker, T., and K. Fessler. 1990. Measles in Milwaukee. *Wis. Med. J.,* 89:403–407.

U.S. Department of Health and Human Services. 1986. *A Report of the Surgeon General: The Health Consequences of Involuntary Smoking. 1986.* Washington, D.C.: U.S. Government Printing Office.

U.S. Department of Health and Human Services. 1988. *A Report of the Surgeon General: The Health Consequences of Smoking: Nicotine Addiction. 1988.* Washington, D.C.: U.S. Government Printing Office.

U.S. Department of Health and Human Services. 1989. *Reducing the Health Consequences of Smoking: 25 Years of Progress. A Report of the Surgeon General, 1989.* Atlanta, GA: Centers for Disease Control, Office on Smoking and Health. DHHS publication no. (CDC) 89-8411.

U.S. Department of Health and Human Services. 1991. *Strategies to Control Tobacco Use in the United States: A Blueprint for Public Health Action in the 1990's.* Washington, D.C.: National Cancer Institute. DHHS publication no. (NIH) 92-3316.

Wynder, E. L., and E. A. Graham. 1950. Tobacco smoking as a possible etiologic factor in bronchiogenic carcinoma. *JAMA,* 143:329–336.

CHAPTER 3

Program Development: A Framework for Health Services

SAM SHAPIRO

Program development often follows a decision that a problem exists and that a solution to the problem must be sought. The topics of problem investigation and problem-solving were considered in the two previous chapters; this chapter extends the discussion into the area of program development.

What needs to be taken into account in developing a program? Are there guidelines that help us make a decision to develop a program and measure its outcome? While "why"and "what are the results" may be stated as simple questions in the initiation of a program, the issues underlying them are complex. This is true when we are concerned with such challenges as the possible modification of the management, organization, and financing of health services directed at cost containment, access to care, utilization of appropriate health services, and health status of a population. To a large extent, the goal of program development in these areas is to identify through the application of epidemiologic methods the interventions that are most promising for favorably affecting health care at acceptable costs.

The approach taken here is to discuss the issues, listed in Table 3-1, and to illustrate how programs related to health services and other areas are identified for development and then conducted.

Policy and Program

Public health policy that states a goal or raises a question about the consequences of an action is frequently the rationale for the development of a program. However, what do we mean by policy and, more particularly, public policy? The literature on this issue is sparse, and there are few examples that can be cited. One that can be given states:

> policy is a set of normative guidelines directed at practice. A public policy is composed of enforceable guidelines, governing a particular area of conduct, that

Table 3-1. Issues in program development

Policy as a forerunner of a program
Factors that influence the development of a program
Utility of evaluating a program
Strength of evidence to adopt a new program
Steps taken to increase the probability of success

have been accepted by an official public body, such as an agency of government or a legislature. The policies of corporations, hospitals, trade groups, and professional societies may have a deep impact on public policy, but their policies are private rather than public. (Beauchamp and Childress, 1994)

Another statement subdivides "policy into two areas: legislation or regulation and organizational policy" (Schmid et al., 1995).

Current examples of public policies include whether health benefits and reimbursement are to be modified under Medicare, whether Medicaid is to move more decisively toward state control, and whether health maintenance organizations and other types of managed care organization are to be promoted by governmental agencies for publicly financed programs. Other examples relate to seat belt laws and smoking in congregate places. The debates in reaching decisions on these issues are shaped by political considerations, with information obtained from past experiences expected to play a role. Programs to implement public policies will be influenced by local circumstances, but the objective will be to create change.

Policies and the development of programs to implement them are most frequently not as far-reaching as those in the public arena. They may be limited to advocacy for a particular component of health care and call for a change in the organization of a care system or in the delivery of a service. This is illustrated by a health care organization's policy to modify its functioning to introduce managed care and improve access to care for vulnerable populations.

What is the primary element that characterizes programs? We may start by defining *programs* as structured interventions designed to implement a policy or to engage in a change dictated by an administrative decision. In essence, a program may be introduced in response to a need after considering alternatives, or it may be adopted on a trial or demonstration basis. Sometimes, political forces form the basis for program development and epidemiologic data may exert a small influence. In any event, evaluation is an essential component of program development, by raising questions that challenge the decision to engage in the program, and special emphasis is given in this chapter to the joint consideration of program development and evaluation.

Development of a Program and Its Evaluation

The process of developing a program may be seen as the systematic assessment of the extent to which the proposed program meets defined objectives or whether specific aspects of a proposed program are superior in costs or effectiveness to those found in an existing program. Implicitly we are saying that a program is initiated when there is reason to question whether change is required in the structure or process of an ongoing program or when a new idea is advanced to enhance the potential for achieving a desirable objective. Judgments may be made about the need for change through information that already exists or that can be developed to clarify the nature of a problem.

The process of developing a program often will indicate the need to provide for evaluation. Uncertainty may have emerged about the choice among alternatives or, for that matter, whether the introduction of a program about which there is little prior knowledge will result in achieving stated objectives. Clearly, there is a need to determine whether a presumably effective intervention leads to the predicted change and, if not, whether the intervention was poorly applied, not generalizable to the type of population being targeted, or inadequate to achieve the benefits expected.

Many states are requiring their Medicaid enrollees to receive their medical care from managed care organizations. The objective is to achieve cost containment at no reduction in access and quality of care. How would a state determine whether this objective is met? A careful assessment would call for information on several indicators before and after the change is made, for example, costs per unit population, rates of immunization of children, and stage of pregnancy when prenatal care begins.

Figure 3-1 describes the activities that integrate the development of programs and evaluation (Shapiro, 1991). This figure shows a loop from information development to the identification of interventions with definable benefits, the evaluation of the persistence of effectiveness, the decision as to whether changes in the intervention should be made, and modifications in the information system to assess the outcome of new changes that are introduced.

Major questions about what is to be addressed in evaluation and the nature of the evidence required face the investigator. A starting point of great consequence is to clarify what is at stake and how ''hard'' the evidence has to be to accept or reject a new measure or to reach a favorable or unfavorable decision regarding an existing program. This depends on a number of issues, such as those shown in Table 3-2.

Closely associated issues relate to the level and nature of the effect. For some problems, it may be adequate to demonstrate that a nontrivial effect, however this may be defined, has been achieved. Many programs, however, require large

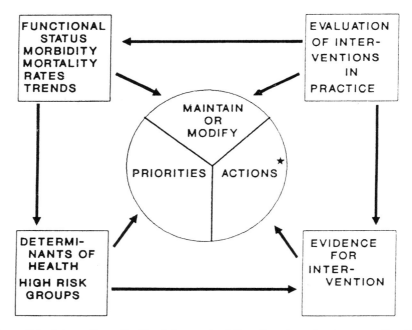

Figure 3-1. Intersections of epidemiology and public policy, from development of health-related information to action and evaluation. *Legislative, regulatory, programmatic.

resources in the implementation stage, and here it is imperative that the intervention have a high probability of causing a change that reaches a level agreed to as consequential.

The "nature of the effect" question brings us face to face with an even more complex issue. For example, are we dealing with a problem that requires measurement of multiple types of outcome that may have different social values, as would be the case if mortality were to decrease but protracted, severe morbidity were to increase? This is the problem that neonatologists face when a very low birth weight baby is born with severe congenital anomalies (Sinclair et al., 1981). Shall all measures be taken to save the infant? Epidemiology can provide information on this question. However, there are also social problems that decision-

Table 3-2. Factors affecting program development

Need for program development seen by planners or administrators
Scope of medical, social, or economic changes sought
Extent of anticipated effect of program
Definition of evaluation phase when planning program
Availability of measures for studies of process or outcome
Acceptability of changes by providers of care and patients

---

makers take into account in resolving this issue, bringing to bear conflicts with the evidence, and in this case, as in other health hazard situations, we have what has been described as "political epidemiology" (Brownlea, 1981).

On another and equally fundamental level, are the indicators of health status widely enough accepted to provide a basis for policy, planning, and administrative purposes? Of considerable importance are the current efforts to go beyond conventional mortality, morbidity, and disability measures. The goal may be to develop scales of social, mental, and physical functioning that provide sensitive measures of health status applicable in determining the effectiveness of health care programs.

With respect to "breadth of the effect," a major issue is whether the intervention may have a significant impact on one segment of the population and not on another. Our knowledge of the etiology of disease and the influence of biologic, social, or demographic factors on the course of illness is so incomplete that frequently one cannot assume that the effect will be the same on all strata of the population. This has led to the insistence of inclusion in research of samples of minority groups and women which are adequate to determine the course of cardiovascular disease. A more specific case is the questionable efficacy of routinely screening women aged 40–49 years for breast cancer (see Chapter 10). Additional research appears to be needed on whether breast cancer behaves differently in premenopausal women from the way it behaves in older women, where the efficacy of mammography has been consistently demonstrated.

Planners, administrators, and evaluators may conclude that appropriate attention has been given to all of the "factors affecting program development." However, the introduction of a program could mean change for which the participation of providers is required, and questions may exist about the acceptability of the program by consumers of health care. The nature and extent of the effort to gain the cooperation of providers will depend on the type of changes projected, but the main point is that the issue is not overlooked. With regard to patients, factors that affect acceptability to participate in the program need to be understood and, at times, negotiations may become necessary. Formal negotiations are unlikely to occur, but again, the point is that consideration of patient response to a change is needed. For example, the closing of a hospital in a community may be justified on economic grounds, but changes in accessibility to services may be the prime question raised by the community, requiring discussion with representatives of the community.

Structuring Program Development and Evaluation

Elements that are important in structuring programs and conducting evaluation are given in Table 3-3 and discussed in the sections that follow.

Table 3-3. Elements of program development and evaluation

Goals, objectives, and underlying assumptions
Operational status of program and population served
Methods projected for evaluation
Potential for implementation of program

Goals, objectives, and underlying assumptions

Identification of the goals, objectives, and underlying assumptions of the program and the subset of components to be investigated can include, as indicated earlier, changes that affect the organization, method of delivery, or scope of services. Here, we are involved with a deceptively simple concept. Determining what is to be evaluated requires an ability to specify clearly the issues and the tools of evaluation, including the measures needed, which must be in a state of readiness for application. While the development of measures or methodologies is essential for advances in the field of evaluation, it is useless to select an issue that requires a new breakthrough in methodology. Further, an extensive time frame runs the risk that conditions in comparative programs will be different at the end of the evaluation from what they were when the evaluation was initiated.

Operational status of the program and population served

By definition, program development consists of an intervention that introduces an activity that had not previously existed. This could take the form of initiating a program in its entirety or of modifying elements that are critical to an existing program. In the latter case, it is important to understand the role that the change is intended to play while maintaining unchanged the rest of the program. For example, immunization programs are not successful in some community groups, and the question is the extent to which the immunization rate will improve if an outreach program is added.

Population characteristics may be related to all in a program or to a targeted subgroup. In addition to demographic variables, population characteristics may include knowledge, compliance, and other health behavioral conditions. A great deal of research has been conducted to indicate the relation of such attributes to utilization of services. However, it is almost always true that maintenance of these characteristics in the evaluation is an essential phase of the analysis of the effectiveness of the change. In fact, when a program is introduced to improve the use of home health care, for example, it would be important to assess the impact of the change in benefits on men and women, racial groups, the financially dependent, and those who have networks of friends and relatives and those who do not.

Methods projected for evaluation

Define the yardsticks and the methodology to be used. Inherent in any evaluation is the need for a comparison with either a widely accepted set of criteria or an
alternative. The criteria may be embedded in the goals or objectives. The alternative may involve contrasting approaches introduced within the program itself or
with other programs from the one being evaluated. How do we choose the
methodology to be applied?

Clearly, the methodology that offers the greatest rigor is the randomized
controlled trial (see Chapter 9), but for many evaluations this may not be feasible.
The design may have to be case-control (see Chapter 8), quasi-experimental
(before and after with a comparison group), or cross-sectional, in which comparisons take into account many of the available variables. Throughout, the concern
is with reaching a decision about the definition of dependent variables that can be
measured reliably and meet criteria of validity. An example of the application of a
quasi-experimental design was the decision to use this method for the evaluation
of a demonstration program in which regionalization of perinatal care for high-
risk pregnancies was introduced in defined communities (McCormick et al.,
1985). Theoretically, the best design for evaluation was a randomized controlled
trial, but this turned out not to be feasible. Instead, nondemonstration areas with
characteristics similar to those of the demonstration areas were followed to see
whether the changes resulted in the hypothesized improvements. The outcome
variables were defined, reductions in low birth weight and infant mortality; and
the source was the vital statistics systems of the areas covered. Another objective
was to determine whether reduced mortality was accompanied by increased frequency of developmental delay and congenital anomalies among the survivors.
Home visits and developmental tests provided the information needed (Shapiro et
al., 1983).

In the development of an evaluation program, another issue to which attention needs to be given is the designation of sample size, and for this there are
well-established statistical procedures to guide us (see Chapter 11). The important point is that we are interested both in reaching a decision about the null
hypothesis with a reasonably high degree of confidence and in reducing the risk of
missing a difference or effect with which we are concerned because of the
inadequacy of the sample size. There are occasions when the evaluation cannot
rigidly adhere to a desirable criterion for sample size. Nevertheless, it is useful to
bear in mind the risk of failing to find an effect because of the relatively small
number of observations available.

Potential for implementation of the program

To determine the potential for implementation of results, evaluation cannot
shoulder the total responsibility for ensuring that action will be based on findings.

Many other factors, including competition for resources, dislocations of existing systems, receptivity, and credibility, clearly may override an unequivocal result. However, evaluation that is preceded by an involvement of administrators, providers, planners, or policymakers in the selection of questions to be investigated and in a commitment to action should substantially affect decisions when the results are available. When change is agreed to, the task becomes one of assessing the extent to which it is applied and whether the effect sought is achieved.

Epidemiology and Its Relationship to Program Development and Evaluation

Embedded in the preceding guidelines are elements drawn from the field of epidemiology, and the remainder of the chapter deals with this area. Health goals and objectives have been adopted as a matter of public policy, with programs to advance health promotion and disease prevention as a central focus through clinical preventive services. It is expected that the effect will be seen in reduced morbidity and improved functional status as well as in cost containment.

Epidemiology has had its most direct impact on program development through the information it has produced on the magnitude of health problems and risk factors and through experimental and observational studies on prevention and control of health conditions. Implementation and evaluation of policies in the form of programs require the participation of other disciplines and close association with public health agencies and systems of health services. The influence of epidemiology at this stage is dependent on increased involvement through which measures of outcome and information on the process of implementation become available. Epidemiologic principles, methodologies, and approaches to assessing evidence are as relevant at this stage as they are in research to determine risk factors and leads to the etiology of disease. This point becomes clear when we consider (1) the approaches to prevention and incorporation of elements into programs through which large gains in improved health are expected and (2) the attention given to increasing the effectiveness of treatment.

The report *Healthy People 2000* (U.S. Department of Health and Human Services, 1991) is encyclopedic, but it gives priorities to conditions that account for the larger share of disability, morbidity, and mortality in the population. As in the case of its predecessor 12 years earlier, *Healthy People, The Surgeon General's Report on Health Promotion and Disease Prevention* (U.S. Public Health Service, 1979), objectives are stated in quantitative terms to measure improvement in a wide range of indicators of health status for the population as a whole and for those who are vulnerable or disadvantaged due to economic, social, and ethnic background; gender; and age. The basic premise of the report is that appropriate application of present knowledge through new programs or enhancing existing programs should result in many of the gains in health status being targeted. For many of the health outcomes, a host of modifications are called for at the individual and institutional levels, with varying difficulties and costs in implementation. Also, frequently, unless provision is made for evaluation, we will be uncertain about the magnitude of the effect of a specific change on a health outcome or costs, and in some cases, there can be a long lag before the targeted improvement can be seen.

For example, we still do not know how to apportion the credit for the substantial reduction in coronary disease mortality during the 1970s and 1980s between prevention requiring behavioral changes to reduce risks (e.g., smoking cessation, lowered blood cholesterol, increased physical activity) and advances in technology and treatment (Havlik and Feinleib, 1979). Availability of this type of information would have mattered in the preparation of *Healthy People 2000* in two ways: it could have guided priorities in allocating resources for program development, and it would have provided a firmer basis for estimating future progress in reducing coronary heart disease mortality.

The continuing difficulty in producing such data is due, in part, to the absence of an established system for tracking trends in the incidence of coronary heart disease and equally, if not more importantly, to the conceptual and methodologic problems in linking behavioral and health care system processes to outcome. The development of models that demonstrate the significance of resolving these issues, along with identifying the data required, would be an important contribution.

Another example illustrates the value of closely monitoring the outcome measure while the intervention is introduced. For years, the case of determining whether the cervical smear (Papanicolaou test) and treatment of cancer of the cervix in situ result in reduced incidence of invasive cervical cancer has been cited as a lost opportunity for definitive study. A randomized trial started 30–40 years ago could have settled the issue long ago, but it is not possible to do so now because of the widespread use of the Papanicolaou smear test (Miller et al., 1976). However, screening programs were started in a few areas, monitoring changes that occurred in rates of in situ and invasive cancers of the cervix and in mortality from this condition. Challenges were common, and it was not until comparative data (areas that had aggressive programs vs. areas that did not) showed a favorable difference that the challenges became less frequent. The point behind this account is not to suggest that a randomized trial is a luxury but that force of circumstance may make it impossible, as for Pap testing, and that other means for reaching conclusions need to be examined.

An example drawn directly from the field of health services research and that has been influenced by epidemiologic principles is the development and adoption of the diagnosis-related groups (DRG) for reimbursement of hospital stays of persons covered by Medicare (U.S. Prospective Payment Assessment Commission, 1990). In this case, a fundamental change in the basis for payment of a stay in the hospital was made from length of stay to reimbursement related to the condition for which the patient was admitted. The mathematical derivation of a formula that separated diagnoses into groups that minimized the variation in costs to hospitals facilitated the introduction of a "per case" payment system. Demonstration programs of various types, but all aiming at cost containment, were carried out in a few states. In 1983, the "per case" scheme was adopted as national policy. Many proposals have been made to modify the formula, and a number have been adopted. The main point is that a method for reducing hospital admissions and length of stays has been in effect for Medicare patients, and this has had the desired effect. Since the introduction of the DRG system of reimbursement for Medicare patients, there has also been a decrease in the rate of hospitalization for all persons, including children.

Aids to Development of Programs and Evaluation

Two activities have had an effect on program development and its evaluation. The first is the *Guide to Clinical Preventive Services* (U.S. Preventive Services Task Force, 1989), a companion volume to *Healthy People 2000*. Its prescriptions for preventive measures reflect the productivity of research and indicate the actions to be taken by clinicians to reduce the burden of disease and disability through screening tests, counseling interventions, immunizations, and chemotherapeutic regimens. Recommendations for a number of widely practiced procedures are being withheld until their benefits are demonstrated through appropriate research. New preventive services that stand the test of efficacy trials or rigorously conducted observational studies are advanced.

Implementing a recommendation from the *Guide to Clinical Preventive Services* can be a complicated affair because of its dependency on decisions that affect more than prevention. For example, counseling by primary care providers to modify patients' health behaviors and life-styles may proceed sporadically unless reimbursement is increased to reflect the additional time required and unless time schedules for seeing patients are restructured. Delay in implementation may occur even where the recommendation is for a well-defined intervention for which the efficacy has been established through randomized controlled trials (see Chapter 9). Breast cancer screening is a recent case that has high public visibility. Access to screening using mammography has been increased by its inclusion in health insurance reimbursement, though for many women out-of-pocket costs for screening remain a barrier. There is evidence, however, that participation by women in periodic screening would increase if primary care physicians more often discussed the desirability of routine mammography screening with their patients.

A second action that moves us from recommendation to program was the establishment of the Agency for Health Care Policy and Research (AHCPR) by the Omnibus Budget Reconciliation Act of 1989 (Agency For Health Care Policy and Research, 1989). This represents one of the policy decisions by the federal government in recent years to support research that can affect medical practices. Many factors accounted for the action taken. In the forefront are past observations that show unexplainable variations across the country in the treatment of specific conditions and the potential for reducing medical care costs through closer examination of the effectiveness of alternative clinical practices. AHCPR has aimed to improve the quality, effectiveness, and appropriateness of medical practice by developing and disseminating scientific information regarding the outcomes of health care services. The agency's program is activist in the sense that practice guidelines and standards are being developed and promoted. As part of the effort to reduce the federal budget, there are now proposals to curtail the functioning of the agency, and further work in this area may become dependent on the initiative of individual researchers seeking support through grants from foundations and government.

Conclusion

When program development in health services is linked to evaluation, we enter an arena that is charged with many of the same requirements present in planning research that has a strong epidemiologic component. The issues we face in structuring the research or evaluation are similar: What are the objectives? What measures can be used that determine outcome? What is the strongest methodology available for the conduct of the study? How are the risks in reaching conclusions reduced?

There are differences, however. The starting point in program development is often a policy decision or an administrative conclusion that a change in financing, organization, or delivery of services is to be introduced. The questions that arise center on the effect of the change on access to care and on the quality and outcome of care. Prior favorable experience with the change could mean that evaluation might be limited to asking whether the change is being implemented in a manner consistent with the expected effects or whether the results call for additional changes.

In carrying out the evaluation, the participation of the key people who are responsible for implementing the results must be obtained. Probing into the circumstances under which prior experience was gained would be useful. For example, the population to which a new application is to be made may differ in its ethnic or economic composition from that of the site from which the information is derived. The issue we face, in the end, is whether we are able to draw conclusions about the generalization of the program's effectiveness.

References

Agency for Health Care Policy and Research (AHCPR). 1989. Omnibus Budget Reconciliation Act of 1989. Public Law 101-239, Title IX, signed December 19, 1989.

Beauchamp, T., and J. Childress, eds. 1994. *Principles of Biomedical Ethics*. New York: Oxford University Press.

Brownlea, A. 1981. From public health to political epidemiology. *Soc. Sci. Med.,* 15D: 57–67.

Havlik, R. J., and M. Feinleib, eds. 1979. *Proceedings of the Conference on the Decline in Coronary Heart Disease Mortality*. Bethesda, MD: National Heart, Lung, and Blood Institute. NHLBI publication no. (NIH) 79-1610.

McCormick, M. C., S. Shapiro, and B. H. Starfield. 1985. The regionalization of perinatal services: summary of the evaluation of a national demonstration program. *JAMA,* 253:799–804.

Miller, A. B., J. Lindsay, and G. B. Hill. 1976. Mortality from cancer of the uterus in Canada and its relationship to screening for cancer of the cervix. *Int. J. Cancer,* 17:602–612.

Schmid, T. L., M. Pratt, and E. Howze. 1995. Policy as intervention: environmental and policy approaches to the prevention of cardiovascular disease. *Am. J. Public Health,* 85:1207–1211.

Shapiro, S. 1991. Epidemiology and public policy. *Am. J. Epidemiol.,* 134:1057–1061.

Shapiro, S., M. C. McCormick, B. H. Starfield, et al. 1983. Changes in infant morbidity associated with decreases in neonatal mortality. *Pediatrics,* 72:408–415.

Sinclair, J. C., G. W. Torrance, M. H. Boyle, et al. 1981. Evaluation of neonatal intensive care programs. *N. Engl. J. Med.,* 305:489–494.

U.S. Department of Health and Human Services. 1991. *Healthy People 2000, National Health Promotion and Disease Prevention Objectives*. Washington, D.C.: U.S. Superintendent of Documents. DHHS publication no. (PHS) 91-50212.

U.S. Preventive Services Task Force. 1989. *Guide to Clinical Preventive Services: An Assessment of the Effectiveness of 169 Interventions: Report of the U.S. Preventive Services Task Force*. Baltimore: Williams & Wilkins.

U.S. Prospective Payment Assessment Commission. 1990. *Medicare Prospective Payment and the American Health Care System: Report to Congress June 1990*. Washington, D.C.: The Commission.

U.S. Public Health Service. 1979. *Healthy People, The Surgeon General's Report on Health Promotion and Disease Prevention*. Washington, D.C.: U.S. Department of Health, Education, and Welfare.

PART II

Epidemiologic
Tools

CHAPTER 4

Management Information in Decision-Making

DONALD M. STEINWACHS

The challenge for management information systems (MIS) in meeting the information needs of health care managers and providers is substantial. The changing health care environment demands new management strategies to ensure organizational survival and to prosper. This chapter focuses on managed care organizations (MCOs) and the MIS role in management decisions regarding the allocation of resources to meet health care needs. The objectives of the chapter are (1) to examine some of the major health care issues facing MCOs, (2) to explore the role of MIS in meeting needs for information to manage care in ways that protect quality and contain costs, and (3) to identify specific MIS strategies for meeting information needs and assessing their state of readiness for implementation.

Initially, some of the management issues facing MCOs are discussed. These include controlling access to and utilization of services, finding new opportunities to improve efficiency, managing quality improvement as an ongoing process, and ensuring that the health care services provided are effective and making a positive difference in patient outcomes. In making these decisions, managers need to understand the decisions made by patients in choosing to seek care and to adhere to provider recommendations, as well as the decisions made by providers in their diagnosis, treatment, and management of patients. To be successful, the manager needs to understand and respond to the expectations of enrollees, payors, regulators, and policymakers.

Issues Faced by Health Care Decision-Makers

The 1990s are proving to be a period of rapid and substantial change in the American health care system. Health maintenance organizations (HMOs) and other forms of managed health care organizations are rapidly growing and becoming the predominant form of health care (Gold et al., 1995). Indemnity insurance is disappearing and is being replaced by capitation payment for the health care for which the enrolled population is eligible.

The stimulus behind the growth of capitation payment and the MCO is being driven largely by rising health care costs. Total health care expenditures are about one trillion dollars per year and represent almost 15% of the gross domestic product. Employers are seeking to control health insurance costs, Congress is looking for savings from Medicare and Medicaid programs, and states are seeking to control their portion of Medicaid expenditures.

The move to MCOs and capitation payment recognizes the strong fiscal incentives under capitation to manage costs within a budget. For MCOs and health care providers, the move to capitation funding is stimulating new requirements for management information that tracks costs, quality, and revenue. For consumers and patients, the focus on cost containment has raised concerns that controlling costs will limit access to care and choice of providers, compromise quality of care, and jeopardize patient outcomes for efficiency. These concerns need to be addressed directly by managers and by the health care industry.

Access to care

Consumers are increasingly concerned that cost containment and managed care will reduce their access to health care. Managers face the question of what is "good" access. *Access* has been defined as the timely receipt of appropriate care (Institute of Medicine, 1993). This definition clearly states the objective of accessible health care. However, the measurement of access is not so clear.

There are no accepted measures of timeliness, yet there are some indicators of delayed care for specific conditions, for example, diagnosis of breast cancer at an advanced stage. The measurement of appropriateness is equally complex. In concept, appropriate care involves services that match the patient's needs and are expected to contribute toward the best achievable outcomes for the patient. In the 1980s, much of the interest in appropriateness criteria centered on the criteria for use of lower cost services when appropriate, for example, substituting ambulatory for inpatient care. More recently, criteria have been developed for judging the appropriateness of specific procedures, for example, cardiac catheterization procedures (Chassin et al., 1987). Appropriateness criteria tend to be applied by payors and MCOs with the objective of reducing the unnecessary use of services. As a result, they do not frequently address the question of whether some people who need care fail to receive appropriate services.

Quality of care and effectiveness

The goal of health care is to provide high-quality care at an affordable price. Quality care is expected to lead to the best achievable health outcomes for patients in a manner consistent with their preferences. As such, concerns with access are central to any assessment of quality, in addition to the choice of diagnostic and treatment processes. Yet when we ask what constitutes effective, high-quality care, the answer may vary with the provider and may not be readily measurable.

There is a long history of the development of quality measurement. In the conceptualization of quality, Donabedian (1982) has focused on three areas: the structure of health care services, the processes of care, and the outcomes of care. The accreditation of health care facilities (e.g., hospitals) by the Joint Commission on Accreditation of Health Care Organizations involves specific criteria related to facilities, staffing, and equipment needed to do surgery or to treat emergency patients. As we have gathered research evidence on the efficacy of specific treatments, it has become possible to identify specific elements that should be present for the quality of care to be judged as high. These elements frequently include tests, patient history, and physical examination findings to support a diagnosis and specific treatments shown to be efficacious in modifying the course (outcomes) associated with the diagnosis.

For example, the diagnosis and treatment of high blood pressure (essential hypertension) are expected to include multiple blood pressure measurements indicating a sustained elevation and choices of treatment consistent with the severity of the elevation that can return blood pressure to acceptable levels. The outcomes involve the prevention of acute stroke and myocardial infarction.

The funding of Patient Outcomes Research Teams (PORTs) by the Agency for Health Care Policy and Research (AHCPR) since 1989 reflects the growing national awareness that better information is needed to understand what care is effective, for whom, under what circumstances, and what types of outcome should be expected (Agency for Health Care Policy and Research, 1989). PORT studies review the scientific literature to assess what is known regarding treatment and outcomes, to use administrative data sources to examine variations in practice and indicators of patient outcomes, and to identify the limits of what is known regarding quality of care. These studies contribute to the development of guidelines designed to identify what constitutes the best clinical practice for specific disorders based on scientific evidence and expert judgment (Chassin, 1993).

Cost and efficiency

One strategy for controlling cost increases is to increase efficiency. This requires an understanding of patterns of treatment, volumes of services, and costs. A common proxy for cost is charges adjusted to approximate costs. However, some studies have found that usual adjustment methods lead to biased results (Trisolini et al., 1987). The mark-up on high-volume–low-cost services may be much greater than the mark-up on low-volume–high-cost services. As a result, managers and providers frequently do not have very precise cost information to guide decision-making. This makes efficiency improvement very uncertain and may lead managers and providers to draw the wrong conclusions regarding sources of efficiency.

Accurate costing of the end products of health care is a long-term objective. It will likely require more precise information on the cost of individual services and better methods for linking the range of services that a patient receives during a single episode of treatment. The purpose would be to determine the cost of treating an episode of a specific condition. Ultimately, MCOs need information on the relation of cost to quality and patient outcomes. This is the information needed by managers and providers to truly manage care, that is, to match the resources to patient needs to achieve the best possible outcomes at an affordable cost.

Management Information Systems

The challenge for MIS in meeting the information needs of health care managers and providers is substantial. As suggested by the range of issues discussed above, the expectations for MIS as the information resource to address these issues could easily overwhelm the capacity to collect and to interpret data on health care delivery and its outcomes. Yet, the changing health care environment demands innovative strategies to respond to cost and quality concerns. Thus, it becomes important to define the boundaries within which MIS can be expected to meet information needs and to examine alternative strategies where information needs are beyond the practical capacities of MIS.

In the following sections, the structure of MIS is discussed along with some of the practical limitations being faced in efforts to expand and extend MIS. The application of MIS to the issues being faced by health care managers is discussed, with a focus on the strengths and limitations of MIS alone and the opportunities for augmenting MIS to overcome limitations. The objective is to clarify the potential MIS role in support of managing care for enrolled populations.

Definition and characteristics

There are many types of MIS in most health care organizations, including medical records, appointment systems, accounting and billing systems, and workload and volume of service reporting systems. Increasingly, there is a need to link multiple systems as a basis for providing information on the full range of concerns discussed above. Ideally, all MIS should share some elements of structure and function; these elements provide the basis for a useful definition:

MIS is a routine and systematic collection of data, integrated into information to support management decision-making. (Steinwachs, 1985, p. 608).

The key words are that the data are "routinely" collected, whether on a periodic sample or on a continuous and comprehensive basis; data are "systematically" collected, meaning that all relevant data elements are captured using the same definitions; data are "integrated" to develop information; and this information is valued for its relevance to "management decision-making."

The question facing many managers is how to enhance existing MIS to provide the information to manage the care of an enrolled population and to control costs. Three issues discussed above—ensuring access, monitoring and assessing quality and effectiveness of services, and cost and efficiency— illustrate some of the issues managers need to address.

MIS used in inpatient and ambulatory care settings should share structural elements. MIS most often collect information at the time of a service event, for example, a patient–provider encounter, hospital discharge, or the ordering of a laboratory test. MIS are expected to capture characteristics of the service event that may include information on the type and quantity of services, charges or costs, and the purpose of the service—for example, treatment of a specific diagnosis. In addition, there need to be two key linkage data elements: a unique identifier for the patient receiving the service and a unique identifier for the provider of the service. These identifiers link separate files that identify and describe the characteristics of the patient and the provider. Using these linkages allows the MIS to profile the total care received by a specific patient or to profile all of the services rendered by a specific provider (Table 4-1).

Missing from this description of MIS is any linkage to information on patient outcomes of care. Unless an outcome is associated with utilization, for example, hospital readmission for a complication of surgery, the structure of MIS around service events precludes capturing information on patients who do not return for services. The assumption that failure to return for care is equivalent to good outcomes has been shown to be highly unreliable. Indeed, patients who are highly dissatisfied with their care may go to other providers or may decide that there is no hope of achieving better outcomes and drop out of care. One of the challenges for future MIS is to develop MIS-based strategies for capturing patient outcomes information and linking it to information on access, quality, and cost. Strategies for linking outcomes information are discussed below.

Access: when is it adequate?

Managing care involves managing access to, and use of, services. This may include access to specific services (e.g., preventive care, routine chronic care management visits, and urgent care), to specific providers of services (e.g.,

Table 4-1. Management information systems structure showing linkage of key elements

Utilization Data	Enrollee File	Provider File
Encounter data	Person ID	Provider ID
Date	Age	Specialty
Provider ID	Sex	Board certification
Patient ID	Address	Location(s)
Source of referral	Dates of enrollment	
Reason for visit	Plan benefits	
Diagnosis		
Tests/procedures		
Treatment(s)		
Referrals		
Disposition/follow-up		
Charges (if applicable)		
Hospital discharge data		
Dates of admission and discharge		
Hospital ID		
Admitting MD		
Patient ID		
Principal diagnosis		
Secondary diagnoses		
Procedures		
Operating MD		
Disposition		
Charges (if applicable)		
Ancillary and pharmacy data		
Procedure/medication		
Date		
Patient ID		
Provider ID		
Test results (optional)		
Charges (if applicable)		

ID, identifier; MD, physician.

specialty providers), and to specific levels of care (e.g., acute hospital care vs. outpatient care). For managed care, controlling access is a means to control unnecessary use or to substitute lower cost services when indicated. At the same time, MCOs need to determine whether the enrollee is satisfied with access arrangements or will likely disenroll from the plan. This is a complex balancing process that requires constant monitoring.

Access to services

Progress has been made in defining timely and appropriate care in several areas. There are accepted guidelines for preventive services that indicate by age and risk status which preventive services are needed (U.S. Department of Health and Human Services, 1991; U.S. Preventive Services Task Force, 1989). Many of these services are captured by MIS that collect a basic data set on each visit and the service provided. What may be missing is information by which to classify risk status, for example, family history. If this were included in enrollment data, it would be possible to profile the preventive services received by each enrollee and to flag those people and services that have not been received on a timely basis.

Chronic disease management is a growing segment of the overall demand for services, reflecting an aging population. In 1990, it was estimated that 61% of U.S. health care expenditures ($425 billion) was spent on the care of chronic conditions (Robert Wood Johnson Foundation, 1995). Questions of access may arise regarding the adequacy of population screening and initial diagnosis, as well as access to continuing management services over time. Applying the principles of tracer conditions for access assessment (Kessner et al., 1973) in the modern context of information systems, MIS can be used to compare estimates of epidemiologic prevalence for hypertension and other chronic conditions with the diagnosed prevalence based on MIS ambulatory care diagnostic data. An example of this in Steinwachs et al. (1995a) points to apparent deficiencies in one MCO related to the underdiagnosis of hypertension in younger adults.

Experience suggests that among those diagnosed and brought under treatment, some may not return for follow-up care. MIS can describe patient patterns of care and flag those not returning within specific windows of time. This capacity provides a basis for the statistical description of risk factors, as well as the opportunity to identify individuals and to directly intervene in their care.

The more uncertain area is the measurement of access for acute problems and symptoms. Early work by Aday et al. (1980) used a symptom response ratio to assess adequacy of access for acute problems. Steinwachs and Yaffe (1978) used two brief questions that were completed by providers at the time of a visit to assess timeliness and need for care. Other indicators have been used, including rates of emergency room visits for nonurgent problems and measures of potentially preventable hospitalizations.

A patient's decision to seek care in response to symptoms initiates a sequence of services that involve cost to the patient and to the health care system. Appropriate care seeking is as important as appropriate system response to a patient's request for care. In part, MCO satisfaction surveys that measure delay in getting appointments and waiting times for care are providing information on patients perceived access for acute problems. One strategy to provide more relevant and sensitive information would be to use the MIS data on visits and diagnoses to stratify samples of enrollees for a periodic satisfaction survey. In particular, MIS could be used to identify enrollees who appear to be at higher risk of having access problems, that is, individuals recently using emergency rooms and urgent care facilities, individuals failing to receive the indicated preventive care, and individuals being hospitalized for potentially preventable reasons.

With the growth in MCOs, there is a growing interest in telephone triage of patient problems and telephone access to medical information as a means to reduce unnecessary visits or as an alternative to a visit. National firms are promoting telephone triage and information services to MCOs as a means to promote appropriate care seeking and reduce ambulatory visits. An MIS linkage that needs to be created is between telephone triage/advice and routine MIS information on visits and other services. In general, MIS have been limited historically in the capture of telephone care contacts with patients: these do not generate patient bills and are not counted in provider productivity profiles. Yet, substantial care is provided by telephone, and there are opportunities to substitute telephone care for more expensive visits. Integration of telephone care contacts into MIS could be an important point of departure in understanding the care-seeking process and in assessing the impact of telephone triage/advice.

Access to levels of care

This is the best developed area of managed care. Appropriateness criteria, such as the Appropriateness Evaluation Protocol (Gertman and Restuccia, 1981; Payne, 1987), have been applied for over a decade. The result has been a substantial decrease in hospital admissions and growth in outpatient diagnostic testing and outpatient surgery. In addition, these criteria linked to financial incentives have led the way to continuing declines in the average length of hospital stays. There has been a parallel growth in home health care and subacute services to provide care and rehabilitation during the recuperative periods following acute care. The criteria being utilized continue to evolve and, in some managed care settings, are routinely captured by MIS. This allows managers and providers to better understand how appropriateness criteria are being applied to enrolled populations and what impact these criteria may be having on patterns of utilization and cost.

Patient outcomes related to access

One of the central questions continues to be when is access good enough? One answer is to examine patient outcomes. One outcome relates to patient satisfaction, which may be reflected in complaints and disenrollment. The National Committee on Quality Assurance (NCQA, 1993) includes in its accreditation standards the use of enrollee satisfaction surveys, as well as management systems for addressing complaints and voluntary disenrollments. So, increasingly, MCOs are collecting satisfaction information. An important step would be the linkage of

MIS information on telephone triage, utilization, and diagnosed morbidity to responses to questions regarding satisfaction with access.

Another strategy for assessing the outcomes of access is through the identification of potentially preventable utilization, such as hospitalization for asthma and diabetic ketoacidosis. These utilization-based indicators of outcome can be developed from MIS hospital discharge abstract data and linked to patient and access characteristics.

There are strategies for addressing outcomes related to access that rely primarily on MIS data alone and those that link MIS and survey data to examine correlates of enrollee-reported access.

Cost control and efficiency: how can they be achieved?

Until the recent growth in capitation payment systems, providers had few incentives to increase efficiency (Steinwachs, 1992). Now, MCOs are searching for best value, value being measured as the ratio of quality to cost. Since measurement of quality is frequently problematic and/or expensive, the focus is frequently on reducing cost. A provider who is more cost competitive can expect to have a greater market share and prosper. Those who are not cost competitive are facing increasingly uncertain futures.

Efficiency is usually measured in terms of costs per unit of output (service) and increases in efficiency as the percentage of reductions in costs per unit of service. At the MCOs or systems level, overall efficiency can be calculated as the cost of all health care services per enrollee per year. To make comparisons across MCO or over time, this ratio needs to be adjusted for case mix characteristics of the enrolled population, using adjustors such as the ambulatory care groups (Weiner et al., 1989).

In this competitive health care market, efficiency improvements are desirable in individual services, in the treatment of episodes of care, and in the long-term management of chronic conditions. The following discussion focuses on the potential role of MIS toward improving efficiency in episodes of care.

Episode of care

One of the interesting methodological problems continues to be the measurement of episodes of care. An *episode of care* can be defined as the set of services received by a patient in response to presenting with a specific problem. If this is an acute problem, the episode is likely time-limited. If this is a chronic problem, care may continue for a lifetime. For practical purposes, this may be divided into annual intervals. Complexities in measuring episodes occur when the patient has multiple health problems, there are reoccurrences of the condition, and the decision rules to link services with episodes are based on partial or incomplete information. For example, linking simply by time interval between services would be expected to be less reliable than linking by time interval and diagnosis or by time interval, diagnosis, and provider assessment of relatedness of the services to a single episode of treatment.

Although there are numerous limitations, the episode framework has proven to be valuable (Hornbrook et al., 1985). It has been used to assess physician requirements nationally (Steinwachs et al., 1986), to examine the response of individuals to alternative insurance coverage (Keeler and Rolph, 1988), and to identify recurrent episodes of mental illness treatment (Kessler et al., 1980), among other applications. The treatment episode is one of the foundations for effectiveness research and for measuring patient outcomes (Grady and Schwartz, 1992).

There are relatively few examples of the application of the episode framework to explicitly examine efficiency. Salkever et al. (1982) used the episode framework to compare cost and outcomes for patients seen by pediatricians and nurse practitioners. This study used observation methods and accounting data to determine costs of provider time, with linkage to MIS to describe the episode of treatment. The results indicated differences in the services received, depending on the type of provider seen initially, as well as cost differences that favored using the nurse practitioner over the pediatrician for the treatment of sore throat and upper respiratory infection. These findings may not generalize across practice settings since patterns of treatment, wages, and other cost factors may vary. The methodology demonstrates a strategy that utilizes MIS linked to other data sources to assess the efficiency of an episode of care.

More recent efficiency improvement efforts use critical path management to identify each step in the treatment process and to ensure that it occurs on time. These methods are frequently targeted to inpatient treatment, where delays in the treatment process may extend the patient's length of stay and substantially increase costs. Again, MIS can be used to describe the range of services received by patients and the approximate sequencing and to assist in the analysis of sources of delays.

Linking cost to quality

The ultimate success of these efforts will be determined by the success in linking efficiency and quality improvements, that is, improving the value of services. Thus, applications of MIS that profile access and quality indicators together with cost are likely to assist managers in targeting their efforts toward areas where greater gains in the value of services can be obtained.

Quality improvement: a continuing challenge

American industry has embraced the principles of continuous quality improvement. These principles come from industrial engineering and the application of quality control methods in industrial and service organizations. Berwick et al. (1991) addressed the fundamental question of whether these quality improvement methods have a role in health care delivery. Their conclusion, and that of others, is a resounding yes.

The quality improvement paradigm is built on principles, information, and problem-solving and -monitoring strategies. The principles focus attention on the need for shared expectations between the provider and consumer (plan enrollee), the critical importance of providing health care of quality, and the recognition that quality failures are costly. One essential element in quality improvement is measurement. To assess quality problems, to understand their causes, and to monitor how solutions are working require that quality be measured. Measurement is the basis for providing quality improvement information and the link to examining the MIS role in quality improvement.

Traditionally, MIS, with the exception of medical records, have not been viewed as having a significant role in quality assessment or quality improvement. The arguments for excluding MIS data have ranged from the lack of clinically meaningful information to challenges that the accuracy of the data was questionable. This is changing. More recently, administrative MIS have sought to obtain more clinically relevant information. In 1991, Medicare introduced diagnosis coding on all physician bills, including office visits and inpatient care. The Health Plan Employer Data Information Set (HEDIS) quality of care data requirements for MCOs are leading to a reexamination of MIS capability to measure quality performance indicators (National Committee For Quality Assurance, 1993). For MIS to be successful will require changes in the coding of some services, the capture of test results for specific services, and data quality monitoring. The current trend is clear: clinically relevant information needs to be integrated into MIS to truly manage health care so that MIS can be a relevant source for population-oriented quality measurement.

Table 4-2 shows a summary of HEDIS 2.0 reporting requirements, with an analysis of some of the potential for capture by MIS. The quality indicators include member satisfaction, process of care indicators, utilzation indicators, the physician network, and financial indicators. Although almost all of these indicators have the potential to be captured by MIS, including accounting systems, there may be special challenges for some MIS. Continuous enrollment (denominator) experience needs to be determined to assess exposure and to calculate the rates of use. For periodic examinations (e.g., mammography), analyses may be

Table 4-2. Health plan employer data information set 2.0 potential of management information systems (MIS) to monitor quality indicators

Indicator	Potential for MIS Capture
Member satisfaction	Low: MIS useful for sampling members for satisfaction survey
Quality/access	
Childhood immunizations	High
Cholesterol screening	High
Mammograms	High
Cervical smears	High
Prenatal care	High
Diabetes: retinal screening	Moderate: need to identify all diabetics
Mental illness: follow-up after hospitalization for major affective disorder	High
Members that visit provider:	
Ages 23–39 years	High
Ages 40–64 years	High
Asthma admission rate	High
Low birth weight rate	High
Physician network	
Physician turnover	High
Board certification	High
Utilization, 9 procedure rates, readmission rate, and overall hospitalization rates	High
Membership/finance	
Members disenrolling	High
Medical loss ratio	High: accounting systems
Administrative loss ratio	High: accounting systems
Revenue requirements	Moderate: derived from accounting projections

Source: National Committee for Quality Assurance, 1993.

limited to a subset of enrollees with specific age characteristics who have been enrolled for a minimum period of time. For calculations of readmission for chemical dependency and follow-up care postdischarge for an affective disorder, index events and follow-up services need to be linked and analyzed. These are all conceptually clear, but the structure of MIS may either facilitate or impede the calculations of these key indicators.

The two critical capacities needed by MIS are to identify denominator enrollment and to link enrollees to the services received, including ambulatory, inpatient, consultant, and emergency services, as well as laboratory tests and surgical procedures. One of the more complex calculations of a denominator population is based on diagnosis (e.g., diabetics screened for retinal problems). This raises questions regarding the accuracy of diagnostic statements and coding. Those persons not diagnosed or in treatment are missed, and those with suspected or ruled-out diabetes are included. MIS strategies are needed to statistically validate the denominator, through linkage to a sample of either medical records or pharmacy records to document the receipt of insulin.

Effectiveness of care: impact on patient outcomes

MIS in health care have traditionally focused on the processes of care, not on the outcomes experienced by patients and enrolled populations. It is generally assumed that improvements in access, quality, and efficiency will lead to better outcomes for patients, as indicated by improvements in the patient's health status (functional status) and satisfaction with the health care received and outcomes experienced. In reality, most providers and payors know little about the outcomes patients are experiencing.

In his 1988 Shattuck Lecture, Ellwood (1988) proposed the concept of a new information system for the purposes of outcomes management. The vision was to routinely capture information on patient outcomes in terms of health status (functional status) and satisfaction to complement routinely collected clinical measures of disease status. This concept has attracted the attention of employers who pay for health care and the MCOs that provide it.

The outcomes measurement paradigm focuses on patients with specific problems/diseases (e.g., asthma) and on those receiving specific procedures or treatments (e.g., cardiac catheterization) (Steinwachs et al., 1994). The ideal data collection strategy is for each patient to complete a questionnaire (or interview) that provides baseline information on health status, satisfaction, and past/current treatment. After an appropriate period of time based on the condition and the treatment, follow-up information is collected on health status, satisfaction, and treatment. The data are statistically analyzed to predict patient outcome status as a function of baseline status, severity, and type of treatment. The expectation is that variations in treatment will be related to variations in outcomes and that more effective treatments can be distinguished from less effective treatments.

Interest in the concept of outcomes management has been sufficient to attract the efforts of a range of organizations, including MCOs. The issues being addressed include (1) the cost and feasibility of capturing patient outcomes information in MCO practices and (2) the utility of the information obtained from analyzing outcomes for application toward improving quality of care and management decision-making.

The Managed Health Care Association has established the Consortium on Outcomes Management Systems (OMS) to test the feasibility and usefulness of OMS for MCOs. The findings from a feasibility study indicated that the participating MCO could capture baseline and outcomes information on chronically ill enrollees identified from MIS sources, such as those with asthma. More difficult and frequently not feasible was the capture of baseline information on patients being scheduled for elective procedures, such as cardiac catheterization. There was insufficient time in the scheduling of cardiac catheterization procedures for questionnaires to be sent to patients and completed prior to the procedure. Without the baseline information, it is not possible to measure changes in health status over the episode of treatment.

The results of the feasibility study were sufficiently promising regarding outcomes for chronic conditions that the group of employers and MCOs has proceeded to testing the utility of outcomes information for adult asthmatics. The baseline survey of 6,645 adult asthmatics in 15 MCOs examined treatment patterns, self-management knowledge, and health status indicators (Steinwachs et al., 1995b). Treatment measures included having a corticosteroid inhaler and using it daily: 74% of severe asthmatics reported having an inhaler but only 57% reported using it daily as recommended. Home peak flow meters are recommended as part of effective self-management. However, only 30% of severe asthmatic patients reported having a home peak flow meter. In terms of self-management knowledge, approximately half of the respondents reported knowing everything they needed to know about what makes their asthma worse and how to avoid it, how to adjust medications when their asthma gets worse, and what to do when a severe flare-up occurs. The interpretation of these findings is that there are opportunities for MCOs to improve quality of care.

The follow-up survey 1 year later provides an opportunity to understand what patient, treatment, and provider factors are predictive of better or worse outcomes. The predictive model of patient outcomes makes it possible to examine the relation between elements of the process of care and patient-reported outcomes. Elements of the process of care for adults with severe asthma include (1) having a corticosteroid inhaler, (2) having a home peak flow meter, and (3) being knowledgeable about the following: how to avoid what makes asthma worse, how to adjust medications when asthma is worse, and what to do when a flare-up occurs. The most consistent findings are that patients who report knowing what they need to know about managing their asthma have better outcomes after 1 year, including fewer asthma symptoms, less frequent asthma attacks, and higher levels of physical functioning and general health (Steinwachs et al., 1995b).

The technology of patient outcomes assessment appears to be promising. If it is to be practical, it needs to be part of an MIS strategy at reasonable cost. The work described above uses MIS to sample patients to be included in outcomes assessment. Other models of outcomes assessment collect limited data from all patients at the time of a visit. Follow-up procedures for patients not returning for care require special data collection efforts. The cost of outcomes assessment is largely driven by the sample size and amount of data collected. The criterion for determining adequacy of sample size and data relates primarily to the ability to make statistical inferences regarding the relation of treatment to patient outcome. Other costs are for analysis and interpretation. As standardized data collection methods and analytic models become more available, these costs should come down.

Discussion

The success of managed health care is likely to lie in its capacity to focus effectively on the following: (1) population needs for care, (2) efficient strategies for meeting these needs, and (3) outcomes assessment to determine how well needs have been met. Routine information is central to each of these three elements.

The MIS field is clearly at an evolutionary turning point. The frame of reference for MIS is turning toward the population at risk, not simply the person who presents for services. To define the population and risks, we need more than age and sex characteristics. At the time of enrollment, patients can provide an expanded set of data that would serve as relevant indicators of the need for care, now not being routinely collected (e.g., preventive care status, chronic diseases, and whether or not receiving care). Visit and services data that are now being routinely captured for administrative uses will need to include more clinically relevant data. This will make it possible for MIS to provide quality performance measures, including HEDIS. One key to accomplishing this objective will be greater integration (i.e., capacity for data linkage) of traditionally separate management and clinical information systems. As this progresses, issues related to the comparability of data items, the accuracy of data, and the protection of patient privacy will demand particular attention in both clinical and management data.

The data collection strategy for MIS will need to evolve in directions that make it feasible to link patient outcomes with data on services received. Levels of linkage that deserve consideration address the following three questions: (1) Has the risk status of the person changed over time, and what relation does this have to needed services? (2) Is access appropriate, and are patient outcomes satisfactory for acute and episodic problems? (3) Is the management of chronic health problems maintaining functional status and quality of life for the patient? Experience suggests that there are efficient strategies to answer these questions.

Linking risk status and services might be achieved through a modestly expanded enrollment questionnaire. Currently, most MCOs know age, sex, and family relationship among enrollees. Not included is information regarding current preventive services status, the presence of chronic diseases, or the presence of health problems for which care is not being received. At annual reenrollment, this information could be updated and lead to statistical comparisons between risk status data and services received during the intervening year. The purposes would be to determine if care matches reported needs and to identify those at higher risk of not having needs met.

Managing acute episodic care requires special attention to access arrangements that include triage and health education functions. Also, the management and outcomes of acute problems need to be assessed. In some organizations, acute care management is being tracked through specialized information systems that use disease-specific care management protocols as a basis for collecting data on each step in the process, including outcomes. The investment in specialized MIS is principally in inpatient, high-cost treatment settings. In ambulatory care, parallel strategies are possible, but they have to be relatively inexpensive and will likely need to integrate the patient's medical record with administrative and quality management data. In several MCOs, investments are being made to develop new ambulatory patient record systems that are expected to better meet the combined needs of clinicians and managers.

Management of chronic diseases involves a longer-term perspective in which health status is likely to vary over time and the treatment focus is on maintaining the highest possible levels of functioning and quality of life. Demands on patients with chronic diseases and on their families are generally substantial and long-term. In particular, the patient and family need to integrate treatment into everyday life and to accept the limitations associated with the disease. The role of managed health care is to ensure appropriate treatment, assist the patient and family in care management, and monitor outcome status. One model for doing this is represented by the work of the Managed Health Care Association Consortium on Outcomes Management Systems described above. Experimentation with this and other models will be needed to collect the information required to truly manage chronic diseases.

In summary, current pressures are to contain health care costs and to ensure that the care provided meets quality and outcomes standards. Both goals require better management information, a population-oriented approach to health care and health status information, and a new level of MIS integration across clinical and administrative functions. Realization of fundamental changes in MIS has the potential to launch us into a new era of health care delivery, where there can be MCO accountability for the total health care of populations and where MCOs can be expected to examine questions related to the efficiency and effectiveness of services on a routine basis.

Many of the issues discussed regarding the growing needs for improved MIS capacity in managed care have a close parallel to MIS needs in public health. Some public health agencies are moving ahead to address these needs by developing new population-based information systems (Land et al., 1995). The MIS capacity is clearly present (Friede et al., 1995), but to be comprehensive, public health MIS will need information that is being captured by MCOs. This is also true for MCOs. For MIS to fully reflect health risks and health care, they will need to extend beyond the limits of medical practice information. This presents a potentially exciting opportunity for MCOs and official public health agencies to collaborate in meeting their joint needs for information.

In moving toward these goals, we must remember that all stakeholders in health care need information relevant to the decisions each has to make: patients need to be able to choose among health plans, payors need to be able to judge the quality of care being purchased and the appropriateness of the price, and public health agencies need to have information by which to hold MCOs accountable and to protect the public interest in their licensing and regulatory functions. MIS that have traditionally been institutional resources to meet internally defined needs for information will increasingly be viewed as a resource for meeting the information needs of all stakeholders, not just those of the provider and manager. This is not too different from expectations of accounting systems, being an accurate source of information on financial performance for stockholders and regulators. The health care challenge is far more complex: the system must account for both its quality and its health status outcomes performance.

References

Aday, L. A., R. Andersen, and G. V. Fleming. 1980. *Health in the U.S.: Equitable for Whom?* Beverly Hills, CA: Sage Publications.

Agency for Health Care Policy and Research (AHCPR). 1989. Public Law 101-239, Title IX, Omnibus Reconciliation Act of 1989, signed December 19, 1989.

Berwick, D. M., A. B. Godfrey, and J. Roessner. 1991. *Curing Health Care: New Strategies for Quality Improvement.* San Francisco: Jossey-Bass.

Chassin, M. R. 1993. Improving quality of care with practice guidelines. *Front. Health Serv. Manage.,* 10:40–44.

Chassin, M. R., J. Kosecoff, R. E. Park, et al. 1987. Does inappropriate use explain geographic variations in the use of health care services? A study of three procedures. *JAMA,* 258:2533–2537.

Donabedian, A. 1982. *Explorations in Quality Assessment and Monitoring: The Criteria and Standards of Quality.* Ann Arbor, MI: Health Administration Press.

Ellwood, P. M. 1988. Shattuck Lecture: Outcomes management: a technology of patient experience. *N. Engl. J. Med.,* 318:1549–1556.

Friede, A., H. L. Blum, and M. McDonald. 1995. Public health informatics: how information-age technology can strengthen public health. *Annu. Rev. Public Health,* 16:239–252.

Gertman, P. M., and J. D. Restuccia. 1981. The appropriateness evaluation protocol: a technique for assessing unnecessary days of hospital care. *Med. Care,* 19:855–871.

Gold, M. R., R. Hurley, T. Lake, et al. 1995. A national survey of the arrangements managed-care plans make with physicians. *N. Engl. J. Med.,* 333:1678–1683.

Grady, M. L., and H. A. Schwartz, eds. 1992. *Summary Report: Medical Effectiveness Research Data Methods.* Rockville, MD: U.S. Public Health Service, Agency for Health Care Policy and Research, AHCPR publication no. 92-0056.

Hornbrook, M. C., A. V. Hurtado, and R. E. Johnson. 1985. Health care episodes: definition, measurement, and use. *Med. Care Rev.,* 42:163–218.

Institute of Medicine, Committee on Monitoring Access to Personal Health Care Services 1993. *Access to Health Care in America,* edited by M. Millman. Washington, D.C.: National Academy Press.

Keeler, E. B., and J. E. Rolph. 1988. The demand for episodes of treatment in the health insurance experiment. *J. Health Econ.,* 7:301–422.

Kessler, L. G., D. M. Steinwachs, and J. R. Hankin. 1980. Episodes of psychiatric utilization. *Med. Care,* 18:1219–1227.

Kessner, D. M., C. E. Kalk, and J. Singer. 1973. Assessing health quality: the case for tracers. *N. Engl. J. Med.,* 288:189–194.

Land, G. H., C. Stokes, N. Hoffman, et al. 1995. Developing an integrated public health information system for Missouri. *J. Public Health Manage. Pract.,* 1:48–56.

National Committee for Quality Assurance (NCQA). 1993. *Health Plan Employer Data and Information Set and Users' Manual,* version 2.0. Washington, D.C.: NCQA.

Payne, S. M. C. 1987. Identifying and managing inappropriate hospital utilization. *Health Serv. Res.,* 22:709–769.

Robert Wood Johnson Foundation (RWJF). 1995. *Annual Report. Cost Containment.* Princeton, NJ: RWJF.

Salkever, D. S., E. A. Skinner, D. M. Steinwachs, et al. 1982. Episode-based efficiency comparisons for physicians and nurse practitioners. *Med. Care,* 20:143–153.

Steinwachs, D. M. 1985. Management information systems: new challenges to meet changing needs. *Med. Care,* 23:607–622.

Steinwachs, D. M. 1992. Redesign of delivery systems to enhance productivity. In: *Improving Health Policy and Management: Nine Critical Research Issues for the 1990s,* edited by S. M. Shortell and U. E. Reinhardt. Ann Arbor, MI: Health Administration Press, pp. 275–310.

Steinwachs, D. M., J. P. Weiner, S. Shapiro, et al. 1986. A comparison of the requirements for primary care physicians in HMOs with projections made by the GMENAC. *N. Engl. J. Med.,* 314:217–222.

Steinwachs, D. M., J. P. Weiner, and S. Shapiro. 1995a. Management information systems and quality. In: *Providing Quality of Care,* 2nd ed., edited by N. Goldfield and D. B. Nash. Ann Arbor, MI: Health Administration Press, pp. 115–128.

Steinwachs, D. M., A. W. Wu, and E.A. Skinner. 1994. How will outcomes management work? *Health Aff. (Millwood),* 14:153–162.

Steinwachs, D. M., A. W. Wu , and E. A. Skinner. 1995b. *Asthma Patient Outcome Project: Report on One Year Patient Follow-Up.* Baltimore: Johns Hopkins University.

Steinwachs, D. M. and R. Yaffe. 1978. Assessing the timeliness of ambulatory medical care. *Am. J. Public Health,* 68:547–556.

Trisolini, M. G., B. J. McNeil, and A. L. Komaroff. 1987. The chemistry laboratory: development of average, fixed, and variable costs for incorporation into a management control system. *Med. Care,* 25:286–297.

U.S. Department of Health and Human Services. 1991. *Healthy People 2000, National Health Promotion and Disease Prevention Objectives.* Washington, D.C.: Superintendent of Documents. DHHS publication no. (PHS) 91-50212.

U.S. Preventive Services Task Force. 1989. *Guide to Clinical Preventive Services: An Assessment of the Effectiveness of 169 Interventions: Report of the U.S. Preventive Services Task Force.* Baltimore: Williams & Wilkins.

Weiner, J. P., B. H. Starfield, D. M. Steinwachs, et al. 1989. Development and application of a population-oriented measure of ambulatory care case-mix. *Med. Care,* 29:452–472.

Chapter 5

Public Health Surveillance and Health Services Research

Stephen B. Thacker
Donna F. Stroup

The effective practice of public health includes surveillance; epidemiologic, behavioral, and laboratory research; outcomes research (including economic analysis and evaluation); and training. Public health surveillance data are used to assess public health status, define public health priorities, evaluate programs, and identify emerging problems and research priorities. In this chapter, we explore the potential uses of health services data in surveillance and the applications of surveillance data to improve health services research. To do this, we first introduce the concepts of public health surveillance and summarize the historical development and applications of this essential public health tool. We then explore previous applications of health services data to surveillance in two case studies and evaluate their usefulness for surveillance. Finally, we discuss future directions in public health surveillance and health services research, addressing special issues such as confidentiality and informatics.

Public health surveillance is the ongoing systematic collection, analysis, and interpretation of outcome-specific data, closely integrated with the timely dissemination of these data to those responsible for preventing and controlling disease or injury (Thacker and Berkelman, 1988). Public health surveillance systems should have the capacity to collect and analyze data (Thacker et al., 1989), disseminate data to public health programs (Langmuir, 1963), and regularly evaluate the effectiveness of the use of the disseminated data (Klaucke et al., 1988). Public health information systems, however, have been defined to include a variety of data sources essential to public health and are often used for surveillance, but they lack some critical elements of surveillance systems (Thacker, 1992). For example, they may not focus on specific outcomes (e.g., vital statistics), are not ongoing (e.g., a onetime or occasional survey), or are not linked directly to public health practices (e.g., insurance claims data).

The history of public health surveillance can be traced to efforts to control the bubonic plague in the fourteenth century and includes such key figures as von

Leibnitz, Graunt, Shattuck, and especially Farr (Thacker and Berkelman, 1992). The modern era of disease surveillance was initiated in the 1950s by Langmuir and colleagues, who focused on the collection, analysis, and dissemination of data on specific diseases to those who need to know (Langmuir, 1963). As later stated by Foege et al. (1976, p. 30):

> The reason for collecting, analyzing, and disseminating information on a disease is to control that disease. Collection and analysis should not be allowed to consume resources if action does not follow.

Unless those who set policy and implement programs have ready access to data, the use is limited to archives and academic pursuits and the material is, therefore, appropriately considered health information rather than surveillance data (Terris, 1992). Thus, the boundary of surveillance practice meets with, but does not extend to, actual research and implementation of intervention programs (Ballard and Duncan, 1994). At the same time, surveillance is more than the collection of reports of health events, and data collected routinely for other purposes may enhance surveillance activities. For example, in 1957, a national weekly influenza surveillance system established by the Centers for Disease Control (CDC) used morbidity and laboratory data from state health departments, school and industrial absenteeism, mortality data from 108 U.S. cities, and acute respiratory illness rates from the National Health Interview Survey (Langmuir, 1987).

Currently, in the United States, surveillance is conducted typically by local and state health departments, as well as by some federal health agencies. Public health practitioners use surveillance for public health application with many health events, including infectious conditions, childhood lead poisoning, leukemia, congenital malformations, abortions, injuries, disabilities and associated secondary conditions, and behavioral risk factors. For example, the National Hospital Discharge Survey, a continuing nationwide sample survey of short-stay hospitals in the United States conducted since 1965 (National Center for Health Statistics, 1977), has been used for ectopic pregnancy surveillance (Goldner et al., 1993) and for surveillance of certain chronic conditions (Higgins and Thom, 1989). In 1981, state health departments began using random telephone dialing for recurrent, cross-sectional, statewide surveys of risk-factor information in cooperation with the CDC's Behavioral Risk Factor Surveillance System (Siegel et al., 1991). State health departments have used information from this system to support personal risk-reduction and disease-prevention activities; for example, the rationale for the New Hampshire Indoor Smoking Act was based on smoking prevalence data from this system (Centers for Disease Control, 1990a). The National Health Interview Survey, which also provides information on risk factors, was used with data from the Behavioral Risk Factor Surveillance System to assess the burden of diabetes mellitus (Centers for Disease Control, 1990b) and to document that coverage levels for U.S. children exceed 95% for the recommended vaccines, among the highest in the world (Centers for Disease Control and Prevention, 1995a).

The registration of all births and deaths, legally mandated in the United States, also contains other health-related information (e.g., birth weight and cause of death) and can be used in monitoring the public's health. For example, the mortality information system provides data (from death certificates) on virtually all deaths and, thus, is extremely useful for assessing the impact of different causes of death and for establishing priorities. Mortality data are regularly available at the local and state levels, and, because of burial laws, mortality statistics can be used at the local level within a matter of days. Mortality data are available on a weekly basis from 121 large U.S. cities as part of a national influenza surveillance system. Maintained and published weekly by the CDC in collaboration with local health jurisdictions, these mortality statistics come from cities that represent about 27% of the nation's population and give a useful, timely index of the extent and impact of influenza at local, state, and national levels (Buffington et al., 1993). The quality of death certificate data may vary a great deal from location to location, from state to state, and particularly from country to country. Physicians' assessments of cause(s) of death are notoriously divergent at times, and even definitions of death, time of death, and words like "infant" are subject to considerable variation. For this reason, comparisons of mortality statistics between time frames and across geopolitical boundaries should be made with extreme caution and only after in-depth knowledge of local customs, changes in coding of death certificates, and advances in medical knowledge, to name some important considerations.

Medical examiners and coroners are excellent sources of data on sudden or unexpected deaths. Data are available at the state or county level and include detailed information about the cause and the nature of death that is unavailable on the death certificate. Data from the national system have been used to investigate the magnitude of the problem of use of methamphetamines, the most widely illegally manufactured, distributed, and abused type of stimulant drug (Greenblatt et al., 1995).

Data collected for other uses can be useful for surveillance. For example, the Medicare system covers hospitalization expenses for about 95% of the elderly population (Health Care Financing Administration, 1989). Caution should be taken in the use of Medicare data for specific outcomes (e.g., cancer) to ensure that coding procedures are accounted for in the analysis (Whittle et al., 1991). Other physician-based systems also provide relevant data (Green et al., 1984). The Food and Drug Administration maintains a system for reporting adverse drug reactions (Faich et al., 1987). Current activities in health maintenance organizations (HMOs) offer opportunities of surveillance activities for defined populations (Durham, 1994). Administrative sources also offer the possibility of surveillance of quality of medical care (Roos et al., 1995).

Use of Public Health Surveillance Data

The structure of a comprehensive modern public health surveillance system is a network of compatible health information systems linked electronically and accessible to public health practitioners on a timely basis (Thacker and Stroup, 1994). Data for the system are collected from many sources, including population-based systems (e.g., the Health Interview Survey or vital records), provider-based systems (e.g., physician, laboratory, hospital records and managed care organizations), payor systems (e.g., Medicare), and administrative records from other entities (e.g., the National Crime Survey of the Department of Justice) (Fig. 5-1) (Thacker and Stroup, 1994). In this distributed data system, four issues become critical: common data elements, timeliness, accessibility, and flexibility. An additional difficulty in putting such a system into operation is that,

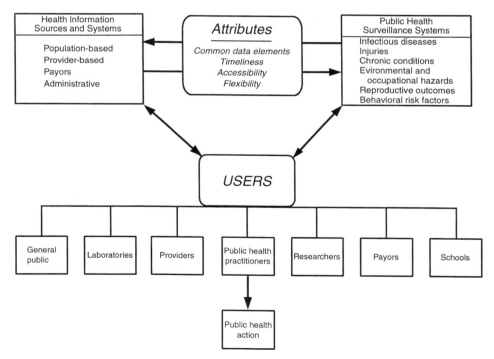

Figure 5-1. A schematic illustration of a comprehensive public health surveillance and health information system.

to work best, it will require a computer system for which only few prototypes now exist (Centers for Disease Control, 1991a). In France, for example, a computer surveillance network that uses present technology has been operating for 10 years and links many physicians throughout the country to a national agency that analyzes and disseminates the data (Graitcer and Thacker, 1986). Indian health authorities are developing an ambitious early warning system, matching cases with clinical disease profiles and laboratory confirmation and linking villages and districts to health information centers via a satellite (Kumar, 1995).

The uses of surveillance information can be viewed in terms of three categories: immediate, annual, and archival (Fig. 5-2) (Thacker and Stroup, 1994). Several recognized uses of surveillance require immediate access. For detecting epidemics, public health officials need a surveillance system allowing access to background data and timely new information. Similarly, for example, detection of unusual clusters of specific birth defects or geographic clusters of pedestrian injuries (Baker, 1989) or detection of a disease in a defined population (Centers for Disease Control, 1995b) is an indication that public health officials should

Immediate detection of:
- epidemics
- newly emerging health problems
- changes in health practices
- changes in antibiotic resistance
- changes in distribution in population

Annual dissemination for:
- estimating magnitude
- assessing control activities
- setting research priorities
- testing hypotheses
- facilitating planning
- monitoring risk factors
- monitoring changes in health practices

Archival information for:
- describing natural history of diseases
- facilitating epidemiologic and laboratory research
- validating use of preliminary data
- setting research priorities

Figure 5-2. Uses of public health surveillance.

respond immediately. For health services, complications of clinical and public health practices, such as mortality associated with the use of insulin-infusion pumps, would require immediate attention (Teutsch et al., 1984).

Besides timeliness after the occurrence of the health event, another aspect is timeliness of access to data when the need arises. For example, an investigator might need background data on previous disease occurrence to evaluate a current report. In this respect, other data sources may enable more timely detection of changes in health practice. An increase in the use of over-the-counter medications, for example, or a decrease in the rate of screening in a group at risk for cervical cancer should signal the need for investigation. The general population's increased use of preventive services recommended for a specific population may be an early clue to the need for public health intervention. For example, an increase in mammography use among young women not necessarily at risk for breast cancer could signal an increase in unnecessary biopsies, with an associated increase in preventable morbidity and cost. Changes in antibiotic resistance patterns may lead physicians to change their prescription practices or researchers to alter their priorities (Centers for Disease Control, 1990d). The recent *Escherichia coli* 0:157 spread among geographically defined populations might have been detected earlier if laboratory data had been linked with physician diagnoses (Centers for Disease Control and Prevention, 1994a).

In the United States, decisions affecting public policy on disease and injury prevention and on allocation of resources to public health are usually made annually with government budgets. Therefore, it is important that policymakers have access to annual data concerning health services. Timely annual data summaries would provide immediate estimates of the magnitude of a health problem, thus helping policymakers to modify priorities and plan intervention programs. These same data would be useful to those assessing control activities and would help researchers to establish priorities in health services research. These data summaries would be even more useful if they were augmented to include complete cost information. For example, beyond the actual costs of the procedure, information on mammography should include costs likely to arise from a positive or negative result (including the cost of a biopsy, treatment for nosocomial infection or other complications, follow-up diagnosis, psychologic stress, and lost work time). Decisions regarding data availability should include careful attention to measures to maintain individual privacy and confidentiality (National Research Council, 1993).

Surveillance data affecting policy or legislation need to be updated annually to facilitate program planning for upcoming years. For example, data showing increases in ambient carbon monoxide levels have led to regulations about the composition of gasoline (Annest et al., 1983). In addition, reviewing surveillance data annually can simplify testing hypotheses related to prevention and intervention efforts. For example, the health effects of increasing taxes on alcoholic beverages can be assessed, in part, by using data on alcohol-associated traffic fatalities.

As intervention programs are evaluated and priorities are set, policymakers must evaluate the effect of the intervention programs on populations. The effect of guidelines and legislation on the use of seat belts or children's safety restraints, for example, can be assessed with data from the Behavioral Risk Factor Surveillance System. Annual monitoring of health practices (e.g., mammography, cervical smears, and cesarean deliveries) and risk factors (e.g., smoking and alcohol use) can provide important clues to the reasons for changes in incidence of related diseases.

Surveillance data should be retained in readily accessible archival form, not only to document the evolving health status of a population but also to help us understand the predictors of disease and injury. These data should be of the best possible quality and should be made available for research, including research outside the government. The integrity of these data must be monitored carefully because previously undiscovered disease patterns may emerge from careful analysis or reanalysis as new analytic tools are applied and as new insights are gained. For example, as we better understand the diffusion of technologies, such as commercial cholesterol tests, more effective prevention strategies may be possible. Carefully maintained archival data can provide an accurate portrayal of the natural history of technology diffusion in a population (Banta et al., 1981). For instance, historical data on mortality attributed to coronary heart disease show that, although coronary heart disease is still at epidemic levels, the rate of such deaths has undergone a decline over the past 25 years (Centers for Disease Control, 1992a).

To measure effectively the long-term effects of public policies or social changes, researchers must have access to archival surveillance and health information systems. For example, the effect of programs to encourage women to stop smoking (Centers for Disease Control and Prevention, 1992b) may be apparent from archival data on lung cancer mortality. In addition, archival surveillance information can be used to validate interim data. An excellent example of a useful surveillance system for policy is provided by the State Cancer Legislative Database of the National Cancer Institute (National Cancer Institute, 1994).

Evaluation of Surveillance Systems

The evaluation of public health surveillance systems is critical to ensuring their usefulness in the allocation of limited resources. The first step in evaluating a public health surveillance system is to describe the public health importance of the event under surveillance (Klaucke et al., 1988). The most important measures to consider for the population under surveillance are the total numbers of cases, both incident and prevalent. In addition, indices of severity, such as mortality and the case-fatality ratio, preventability of the outcome, and measures of functional impairment, are important for surveillance. In the health services research context, an evaluation should consider also intermediate outcomes (e.g., control of hypertension) that are incontrovertibly linked to outcomes (e.g., stroke). The description of the surveillance system should include objectives, case definitions, and the specific components of data collection, analysis, and dissemination. Most important, the usefulness of the system should be presented as the actions taken and the results obtained, based on the data.

Subsequently, an evaluation of a surveillance system includes assessment of system attributes. Is the system sufficiently simple to be usable, or is it so complex as to impede public health intervention? Is the system flexible (i.e., can it adapt to changing disease characteristics and population structures)? Is the system acceptable to both data collectors and users? Is the burden on the data provider minimized?

More quantitative attributes to be evaluated include sensitivity, positive predictive value, representativeness, and timeliness. A sensitive system is very important in detecting acute events for intervention. However, high sensitivity comes at a cost (e.g., increased false-positives), and this attribute may be less important for other uses. However, the positive predictive value of a system is important to reduce inefficient uses of resources (see Chapter 10).

The system should represent the population under consideration not only as to demographics and geography but also as to the appropriate time period under investigation. Historical data may not be helpful in addressing current health problems affected by shifting demographic patterns or changes in case definitions. In addition, timeliness depends on the intended use of the data. Rapid dissemination of data is needed to address acute outbreaks of communicable diseases; however, justifying annual budgets or monitoring long-term patterns of illness typically requires less timely data. Finally, a cost analysis of the system should delineate the resources used to operate the entire system, including costs incurred by providers, insurers, and other elements of the health services activity (e.g., standardizing reporting formats for clinical data).

Case studies

Notifiable disease surveillance

Surveillance for notifiable conditions in the United States is done through the National Notifiable Diseases Surveillance System, which illustrates the use of health services data for public health surveillance. Each state determines its own list of notifiable conditions and mandates that health care providers report these conditions to local and state health departments. The national system relies on consensus, cooperation among states, and technical assistance from national surveillance staff rather than on national directives or legislation.

Since 1989, data on these notifiable conditions have been transmitted electronically from each state health department to the CDC weekly through the National Electronic Telecommunications System for Surveillance (NETSS) (Centers for Disease Control, 1991b). The data are disseminated in the *Morbidity and Mortality Weekly Report*, the *Summary of Notifiable Diseases*, and special reports (e.g., Farley et al., 1992). The reporting format for NETSS allows inclusion of disease-specific information (besides a core record common to all conditions) and early, provisional reporting with subsequent capacity for updating.

In some states, reporting from public health laboratories is automated through the Public Health Laboratory Information System (Bean et al., 1991), which, in these states, is integrated with the NETSS (Centers for Disease Control, 1991c). As part of a current immunization effort in the United States, expanded surveillance for vaccine-preventable diseases is being done using the technologic capabilities of the NETSS, thereby reducing the need for this supplemental surveillance (Centers for Disease Control and Prevention, 1994b).

Data from notifiable disease systems have been used at the local level to document the effect of immunization efforts, such as the downward trend in measles (Centers for Disease Control and Prevention, 1994c) (Fig. 5-3), to demonstrate public health need (Thacker, 1991) or to detect outbreaks (Stroup et al., 1993). At a national level, the data are used more often to monitor the natural history of a condition (Centers for Disease Control, 1992a) or to detect changes in health practice (Cowan et al., 1993). Examination of routinely collected data from contiguous states reveals that infectious diseases, such as salmonellosis, cross state boundaries (Fig. 5-4).

Question 1*. For this case study, are the sources of the data described? Is the burden on the data provider minimized?*

State health departments receive reports from county/local health departments, which receive reports from health providers. In turn, state health departments provide data for the National Notifiable Diseases Surveillance System. This national system uses an electronic format, which is compatible with the laboratory system and which reduces the need for duplicate reporting systems. In addition, the CDC offers technical assistance to the state health departments so that the system for national reporting also helps local public health practice.

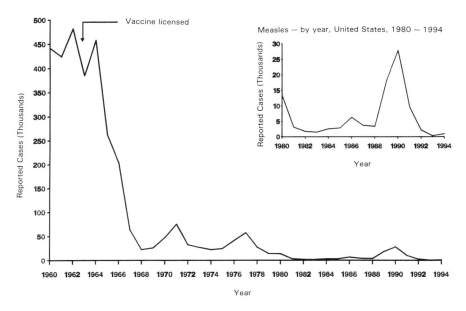

Figure 5-3. Reported Cases of Measles by Year, United States, 1960–1994.

Question 2. *Comment on the timeliness and sensitivity of the system.*

The system is extremely timely at the national level: data reported to the CDC are published in the *Morbidity and Mortality Weekly Report* and available on CDC programs within a week of report. Other lags (e.g., county to state or health care provider to local health department) may be less timely due to lack of funding. Because the data are provisional and often underreported, the sensitivity may be low. However, the ability of the system to accept updated records and an annual review of the data enhance the ability of the system to detect cases.

Question 3. *How could one assess the cost of this system?*

Costs should be assessed at each level. At the national level, costs should include direct costs (e.g., personnel, equipment, and computer time). Although no direct funding is given to states for this surveillance activity, system development and technical assistance at the national level are important in the system's capacity. Additionally, societal costs will include productivity costs (e.g., lost work time due to preventable illness).

Questions for the Reader. *In the development of systems for health reform activities in states, assess the contribution of the notifiable disease system* *to public health. What are some limitations of this system? How could additional data sources be used to address these limitations? What recommendations would you make for improved utility of the system for health services research?*

Breast cancer surveillance

To aid planning and to facilitate evaluation of national breast cancer programs, trends in both incidence and mortality for breast cancer were monitored from 1973 to 1987 (Qualters et al., 1992). Deaths from breast cancer were identified from the CDC's public use files using underlying cause of death (Centers for Disease Control, 1991d). Denominators for rate calculations were obtained using intercensal estimates. Analyses were done for the total female population, as well as for white women and black women. Analyses by race, state, and calendar year

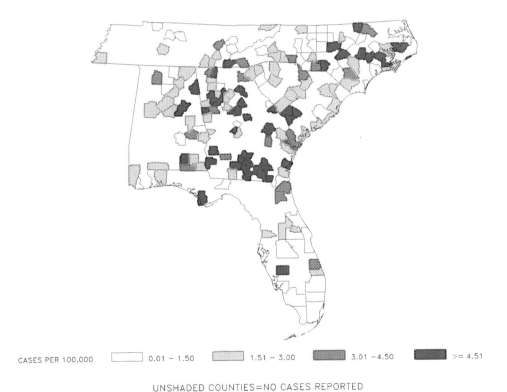

CASES PER 100,000   ☐ 0.01 – 1.50   ▨ 1.51 – 3.00   ▨ 3.01 – 4.50   ■ >= 4.51

UNSHADED COUNTIES=NO CASES REPORTED

Figure 5-4. Salmonellosis rates by county, Georgis and contiguous National Electronic Telecommunications Systems for Surveillance (NETSS) states.

as well as age-specific mortality rates were presented. For a few analyses, data from several calendar years were combined to increase precision.

Incidence data were obtained from public use tapes provided by the Surveillance, Epidemiology, and End Results (SEER) program of the National Cancer Institute (Reis et al., 1991). Breast cancer cases were defined as tumors with primary sites with specified International Classification of Diseases (ICD) codes. Population estimates for the geographic areas covered by the National Cancer Institute were from the U.S. Department of the Census. Both age-specific and age-adjusted incidence rates were calculated for invasive disease; the stage of diagnosis was also examined.

Whereas breast cancer mortality remained stable during the surveillance period, incidence increased during the 1980s. Incidence increased with age, though mortality was constant (Fig. 5-5). Overall, white women experienced lower overall mortality rates for breast cancer than did black women (27.1 vs. 30.3 per 100,000 women in 1987); however, the differences between whites and blacks varied by age (Fig. 5-6). While overall mortality for white women has been stable since 1980, small increases in mortality have occurred in white women more than 60 years of age. Black women more than 60 years of age exhibited higher increases in mortality over time than did white women in comparable age groups. The incidence of in situ and localized cancer showed an increase in the 1980s (Fig. 5-7), which may correspond to increased use of mam-

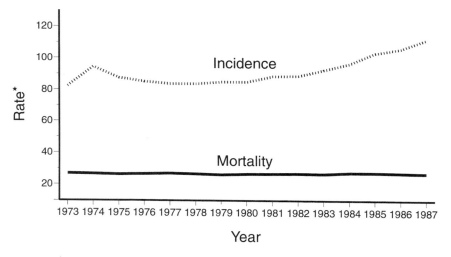

* Cases per 100,000 women.

Figure 5-5. Trend in breast cancer morbidity and mortality, United States, 1973–1987. Source: SEER = Surveillance, Epidemiology, End Results Program, National Cancer Institute.

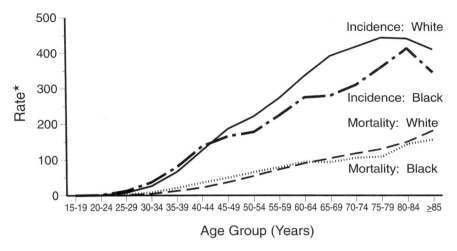

* Cases per 100,000 women.

Figure 5-6. Breast cancer mortality by race and age, United States, 1973–1987. Source: Seer = Surveillance, Epidemiology, End Results Program, National Cancer Institute.

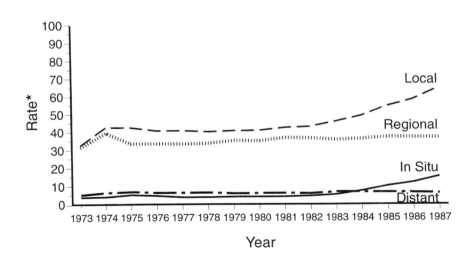

* Cases per 100,000 women.

Figure 5-7. Breast cancer by type, United States, 1973–1987. Source: Seer = Surveillance, Epidemiology, End Results Program, National Cancer Institute.

mography. The rates in this report may be biased because of differences in case findings and case definitions over time (Qualters et al., 1992). Mortality rates are affected by the accuracy of death certificates, and no attempt was made in the analyses presented to adjust for these potential sources of bias.

For women 50–70 years of age, the benefits of mammography combined with clinical breast examination are well known and the value of screening is widely accepted (Fletcher et al., 1993). Improved survival results from early diagnosis and treatment of breast cancer show that there is an 83% 5-year survival for all stages of invasive breast cancer (all women) and a 96% 5-year survival for localized breast cancer (Kosary et al., 1995). Survival increases dramatically with malignancies diagnosed at an early stage.

Current racial differences in mortality may be explained in part by differences in stage of disease at diagnosis and differences in stage-specific survival (Eley et al., 1994) . These data also document that black women have a poorer survival experience with cancer. Despite increasing frequency of screening and improvements in management, more than 43,000 women died of breast cancer in 1992.

> *Question 1. Did the authors describe the public health importance of breast cancer? What data sources were used?*

The authors showed that breast cancer is the most commonly diagnosed cancer and second leading cause of cancer death among women in the United States. They also showed that breast cancer screening is effective in preventing mortality. The authors gave a brief description of the data sources, which were public use files compiled by the CDC and the National Cancer Institute.

> *Question 2. Are these data useful?*

Because of the importance of this problem and the need for assessing ongoing intervention activities, these data are very important in assessing the effectiveness of a public health intervention. In addition, the data may lead to a reassessment of current age-appropriate recommendations for mammography utilization (e.g., leading to recommendations for additional clinical trials) (Eddy et al., 1988). These surveillance data could be used to show stage-specific survival by treatment and race or age. The surveillance data do not address directly some issues, such as biologic differences in tumors and populations or changes in treatment or diagnosis. For health services research, data on services (e.g., mammography, biopsies, and treatment) should be linked to these surveillance data.

> *Question 3. Using the standard evaluation attributes for public health surveillance, how would you characterize the system?*

The system is relatively simple because it uses information already collected by the CDC and there is some flexibility in the system as the ICD codes are modified.

However, there is limited information available on the death certificate and revision is not timely. In addition, since ICD codes generally are grouped by organ systems for publication purposes, recoding may be necessary for surveillance use.

The sensitivity and representativeness of death certification in detecting breast cancer mortality are quite good, yet the representativeness of the SEER data is limited by geographic distribution. The SEER registries cover about 10% of the U.S. population but are not statistical samples. The positive predictive value is not clear, and additional data would need to be collected to assess this.

As noted above, CDC data for mortality contain essentially all deaths in the total population, though there may be biases in coding that affect geographic or race/ethnic data. Data from mortality statistics are generally available at the national level 2–3 years after the year of death. At the local level, these data are more readily accessible. Similar lag times exist for the SEER data, to ensure their accuracy, completeness, and validity.

Question 4. How could the costs of these systems be determined?

Costs could be estimated from the CDC and the National Cancer Institute data. Because these data are collected already and analyzed to a limited degree, the costs of additional use for surveillance are probably relatively small. Developmental and maintenance costs of both of the systems, however, are quite large.

Questions for the reader. How would you assess this surveillance system as to public health needs for morbidity and mortality data? Are the data sufficiently accurate and unbiased? What recommendations would you make for improving the system? What additional data would be helpful in assessing programs? Are the data sufficiently timely for intervention and other public health needs?

Confidentiality

In the conflict between an individual's right to privacy and the general community's welfare, our society has generally favored the rights of the individual. An exception to this in public health is the policy of involuntary isolation for people who refuse to follow physicians' recommendations for diseases of serious public health risk, most recently those with multidrug-resistant tuberculosis. While the risks of major or deliberate violations of privacy or confidentiality are extremely low in public health surveillance systems, there is a danger that violations not involving surveillance data bases can engender public indignation and have damaging spillover effects on public health programs. While we must do all we can to ensure that any national surveillance system is not intrusive and that individual privacy is guarded (Committee on National Statistics, 1993), we as a society must make a larger commitment to ensuring that health information on individuals is available to public health practitioners so that they can implement a more useful system of public health surveillance (Gostin et al., 1993).

Advances in Science

Scientific study and the practice of public health surveillance have a synergistic relation. On the one hand, surveillance data have been used to stimulate epidemiologic and laboratory research (Mulinare et al., 1988; Centers for Disease Control, 1990d). On the other hand, the practice of public health surveillance has been enhanced by contributions from various scientific disciplines, including epidemiology, mathematics and statistics, information sciences, laboratory sciences, behavioral sciences, and clinical medicine (Kilbourne, 1992; Reynolds et al., 1989; Dean et al., 1993).

We can expect further developments in these areas. Epidemiologists will define more precisely risk factors for disease and injury. We will learn, for example, preventable risk factors for conditions and outcomes ranging from obesity to homicide, and this knowledge will be used to target prevention activities. As data in physicians' offices become available through access to computerized patient records, statistical tools integrated into user-friendly computer networks will make a large volume of data rapidly available to all levels of public health. Laboratories will make enormous advances in their ability to link risk with disease outcome through biologic markers of exposure (Centers for Disease Control, 1988). Findings from the behavioral sciences will be incorporated routinely into public health practice as we attempt to reduce people's risk of acute and chronic diseases and injury (Kachur, 1996). We should generate hypotheses, for example, on how to measure true risk factors more precisely in populations (Centers for Disease Control, 1993).

Findings from other scientific disciplines also will contribute to effective public health surveillance. For example, statisticians have contributed to the science of forecasting future trends using surveillance information (Choi and Thacker, 1981), and economic analyses have enhanced our ability to evaluate the impact of prevention (Gorsky and Teutsch, 1995). Not only must public health scientists be open to potential contributions from a variety of established disciplines, but we must also seek out contributions from currently unexplored disciplines.

Conclusion

To develop a comprehensive approach to public health surveillance and health information, several steps are necessary. First, we must strengthen the utility of existing surveillance and health information networks. To do this, those involved in the implementation of this comprehensive approach must recognize that provisional data are sometimes essential for timely action. In addition, whenever we use data for surveillance from a system designed for other purposes, we may need to modify that system to ensure usefulness. While such activities may require a significant change in current practice, development of practical, comprehensive systems of public health surveillance and health information is necessary to equip public health practioners with the tools necessary to meet the challenges of health care reform, information technology development, and the growth of information in private industry.

Second, we may need new sources of data, where no current system is readily adaptable. At any level in the health care system, the most timely and accurate sources of such data are clinicians. The use of sentinel physician practices for surveillance of problems defined by geography or specialty in the U.S. experience has been limited (Centers for Disease Control and Prevention, 1995b). Rigorous assessment and true integration into public health practice are lacking, however. Networks of sentinel clinical practices in France, Belgium, and Great Britain have been integrated into public health practice. In the development of data systems for the United States, the traditional surveillance of disease and injury must be linked to the data sources of managed care. In the development of regional and national networks to serve the needs of consumers, practitioners, health plans, and health alliances, the government agencies responsible for protecting the health of communities must be involved.

Third, we must combine data from many sources, including health services data (Williamson et al., 1994). Although confidentiality and other legal considerations may preclude exact linkage, consensus on uniform data elements is critical. Efforts toward this goal have begun in data collection for both infectious and chronic diseases. Besides expanding data collection, we must discuss problems related to both data analysis and dissemination (e.g., cost).

In the United States, a sociologic trend is shifting in the health care industry, from one dominated by a large number of small offices to one characterized by a small number of large managed care organizations with computerized patient records. As part of this trend, new data systems offer opportunities to public health for prevention. For example, as of June 1995, 32% of Medicaid beneficiaries were enrolled in managed care organizations compared with 14% in 1994. Furthermore, historically HMOs have included prevention as they have developed systems to measure performance and quality of service. One example of an internal performance-measurement and quality-improvement system is the "report card" known as the Health Plan Employer Data and Information Set (HEDIS) (National Committee for Quality Assurance, 1993). Several of the indicators are preventive: incidence of low birth weight infants, utilization of

vaccinations, mammography, cervical cancer screening, screening for cholesterol, prenatal care, and retinal examinations for persons with diabetes (National
Committee for Quality Assurance, 1995). Public health, however, will continue
to require multiple sources of data to accomplish its mission: reports of health
events affecting individuals; vital statistics on the population; information on the
health status, risk behaviors, and experiences of populations; information on
potential exposure to environmental agents; information on existing public health
programs; information from other organizations (e.g., transportation and law
enforcement); and information on the health care system.

A distributed system of coordinated, timely, and useful multisource public
health surveillance and health information data can be developed. Similar systems are used today in finance, travel, and retail marketing, but no such system is
used routinely in public health practice in the United States. The technology and
many necessary data are available (Van Grevenhof et al., 1991). To make these
useful, our society must have a sufficient commitment to develop and maintain
such a distributed system for public health. This commitment must be under-
scored by the recognition and acceptance of the needs for both community health
and individual confidentiality.

Only when individuals in society recognize the link between good public
health data and the prevention of unnecessary disease and disability will public
health information systems be comparable with information systems used in
industry. Educating people about the advantages of having a comprehensive
public health surveillance and health information system is a major public health
challenge of this decade.

References

Annest, J. L., J. L. Pirkle, D. Makuc, J. W. Neese, et al. 1983. Chronological trend in
    blood lead levels between 1976 and 1980. *N. Engl. J. Med.*, 308:1374–1377.
Baker, E. L. 1989. Sentinel event notification system for occupational risks (SENSOR):
    the concept. *Am. J. Public Health,* 79(suppl.):18–20.
Ballard, D. J., and P. W. Duncan. 1994. Role of population-based epidemiologic surveil-
    lance in clinical practice guideline development. In: *Methodology Perspectives,*
    edited by K. A. McCormick, S. R. Moore, and R. A. Siegel. Washington, D.C.:
    U.S. Department of Health and Human Services, Public Health Service, Agency
    for Health Care Policy and Research. AHCPR publication no. 95-0009.
Banta, H. D., C. V. Behney, and J. S. Willems. 1981. *Toward Rational Technology in
    Medicine.* New York: Springer.
Bean, N. H., S. M. Martin, and H. Bradford. 1991. PHLIS: an electronic system for
    reporting public health data from remote sites. *Am. J. Public Health,* 89:1273–
    1276.
Buffington, J., L. E. Chapman, L. M. Chapman, et al. 1993. Do family physicians make
    good sentinels for influenza? *Arch. Fam. Med.,* 2:859–864.

Centers for Disease Control. 1988. Serum 2,3,7,8-tetrachlorodibenzo-p-dioxin levels in US Army Vietnam-era veterans. The Centers for Disease Control Veterans Health Studies. *JAMA*, 260:1249–1254.

Centers for Disease Control, 1990a. State coalitions for prevention and control of tobacco use. *Morb. Mortal. Wkly. Rep.*, 39:476, 483–485.

Centers for Disease Control, 1990b. Regional variation in diabetes mellitus prevalence— United States, 1988 and 1989. *Morb. Mortal. Wkly. Rep.*, 39:805–809.

Centers for Disease Control. 1990c. Update: *Salmonella enteritidis* infections and shell eggs United States, 1990. *Morb. Mortal. Wkly. Rep.*, 39:909–912.

Centers for Disease Control. 1990d. Plasmid-mediated antimicrobial resistance in *Neisseria gonorrhoeae*—United States, 1988 and 1989. *Morb. Mortal Wkly. Rep.*, 39:284–287, 293.

Centers for Disease Control. 1991a. *Wide-Ranging On-Line Data for Epidemiologic Research*. Atlanta, GA: WONDER.

Centers for Disease Control. 1991b. National Electronic Telecommunications system for Surveillance—United States, 1990–1991. *Morb. Mortal. Wkly. Rep.*, 40:502– 503.

Centers for Disease Control. 1991c. *Surveillance Coordination Group Report: Recommendations on Electronic Systems for Public Health Surveillance*. Atlanta, GA: Centers for Disease Control.

Centers for Disease Control. 1991d. *Vital Statistics Mortality Data, Multiple Causes of Death, 1973–80, 1981 and 1982, 1983–87* (Machine-readable public use tapes). Hyattsville, MD: U.S. Department of Health and Human Services, Public Health Service, CDC.

Centers for Disease Control and Prevention. 1992a. *Health United States*. Hyattsville, MD: U.S. Department of Health and Human Services.

Centers for Disease Control and Prevention. 1992b. Cigarette smoking among adults— United States, 1990. *Morb. Mortal. Wkly. Rep.*, 41:354–355, 361–362.

Centers for Disease Control and Prevention, 1993. Use of race and ethnicity in public health surveillance. Summary of the DC/ATSDR workshop. Atlanta, Georgia, March 1-2, 1993. *Morb. Mortal. Wkly. Rep.*, 42:1–16.

Centers for Disease Control and Prevention. 1994a. Foodborne outbreaks of enterotoxigenic *Escherichia coli*—Rhode Island and New Hampshire 1993. *Morb. Mortal. Wkly. Rep.*, 43:81, 87–89.

Centers for Disease Control and Prevention. 1994b. Monthly immunization table. *Morb. Mortal. Wkly. Rep.*, 43:403.

Centers for Disease Control and Prevention. 1994c. Summary of notifiable diseases. *Morb. Mortal. Wkly. Rep.*, 43:50.

Centers for Disease Control and Prevention. 1995a. Vaccination coverage of 2-year-old children—United States, January–March, 1994. *Morb. Mortal. Wkly. Rep.*, 44:142–143, 149–150.

Centers for Disease Control and Prevention. 1995b. Occupational silicosis—Ohio, 1989– 1994. *Morb. Mortal. Wkly. Rep.*, 44:61–64.

Choi, K., and S. B. Thacker. 1981. An evaluation of influenza mortality surveillance, 1962–1979. 1. Time series forecasts of expected pneumonia and influenza deaths. *Am. J. Epidemiol.*, 113:215–226.

Committee on National Statistics, Commission on Behavioral and Social Sciences and Education, National Research Council, Social Science Research Council. 1993.

Private Lives and Public Policies: Confidentiality and Accessibility of Government Statistics, edited by G. T. Duncan, T. B. Jagine, V. A. de Wolfe. Washington, D.C.: National Academy Press.

Cowan, L. D., M. R. Griffin, C. P. Howson, et al. 1993. Acute encephalopathy and chronic neurological damage after pertussis vaccine. *Vaccine,* 11:1371–1379.

Dean, A. G., J. A. Dean , J. H. Burton, et al. 1993. A Word Processing, Database, and Statistics Program for Epidemiology on Microcomputers Computer Program. Epi Info, Version 6. Atlanta, GA.: Centers for Disease Control and Prevention.

Durham, M. L. 1994. Prospects and problems in using data from HMOs for the study of aging populations and their health care needs. *Gerontologist,* 34:481–485.

Eddy, D. M., V. Hasselblad , W. McGivney, et al. 1988. The value of mammography screening in women under age 50 years. *JAMA,* 259:1512–1519.

Eley, J. W., H. A. Hill, V. W. Chen, et al. 1994. Racial difference in survival from breast cancer: results of the National Cancer Institute black/white cancer survival study. *JAMA,* 272:947–954.

Faich, G. A., D. Knapp, M. Dreis, et al. 1987. National adverse drug reaction surveillance—1985. *JAMA,* 257:2068–2070.

Farley, M. M., D. S. Stephens, P. S. Brachman, Jr., R.C. Harvey , et al. 1992. Invasive *Haemophilus influenzae* disease in adults: a prospective population-based surveillance. *Ann. Intern. Med.,* 116:806–812.

Fletcher S. W., W. Black , R. Harris , B. K. Rimer, and S. Shapiro 1993. Report of the International Workshop on Screening for Breast Cancer. *J. Natl. Cancer Inst.,* 85:1644–1656.

Foege, W. H., R. C. Hogan, and L. H. Newton. 1976. Surveillance projects for selected diseases. *Int. J. Epidemiol.,* 5:29–37.

Goldner, T. E., H. W. Lawson, Z. Xia, and H. K. Atrash. 1993. Surveillance for ectopic pregnancy—United States, 1970–1989. *Morb. Mortal. Wkly. Rep.,* 42:73–85.

Gorsky, R. D. and S. M. Teutsch, 1995. Assessing the effectiveness of disease and injury prevention programs. *Morb. Mortal. Wkly. Rep.,* 44: 1–12.

Gostin, L. O., J. Turek-Brezina, M. Powers, et al. 1993. Privacy and security of personal information in a new health care system. *JAMA,* 270:2487–2493.

Graitcer, P. L., and S. B. Thacker. 1986. The French connection. *Am. J. Public Health,* 76:1285–1286.

Green, L. A., M. Wood, L. Becker, et al. 1984. The ambulatory sentinel practice network: purposes, methods, and policies. *J. Fam. Pract.,* 18:275–280.

Greenblatt, J. C., J. C. Gfroerer and D. Melnick. 1995. Increasing morbidity and mortality associated with abuse of methamphetamine—United States, 1991–1994. *Morb. Mortal. Wkly. Rep.,* 44:882–886.

Health Care Financing Administration. 1989. *Medicare Enrollment, 1986–87.* Baltimore: U.S. Department of Health and Human Services. HCFA publication no. 03282.

Higgins, M., and T. Thom. 1989. Trends in CHD in the United States. *Int. J. Epidemiol.* 18(suppl. 1):S58–S66.

Kachur, P. 1996. School-associated violent deaths in the United States, 1992–1994. *JAMA,* 275:1729–1733.

Kilbourne, E. M. 1992. Informatics in public health surveillance: current issues and future perspectives. *Morb. Mortal. Wkly. Rep.,* 41(suppl.):91–99.

Klaucke, D. N., J. W. Buehler, S. B. Thacker, et al. 1988. Guidelines for evaluating surveillance systems. *Morb. Mortal. Wkly. Rep.,* 37(suppl. 5):1–18.

Kosary, C. L., L. A. G. Ries, B. A. Miller, et al. 1995. *Tables and Graphs.* Bethesda, MD: National Cancer Institute. NIH publication no. 96-2789.

Kumar, S. 1995. India's early warning system for epidemics. *Lancet,* 345:917.

Langmuir, A. D. 1963. The surveillance of communicable diseases of national importance. *N. Engl. J. Med.,* 288:182–192.

Langmuir, A. D. 1987. The territory of epidemiology: pentimento. *J. Infect. Dis.,* 155:349.

Mulinare, J., J. F. Cordero, J. D. Erickson, et al. 1988. Periconceptual use of multivitamins and the occurrence of neural tube defects. *JAMA,* 260:3141–3145.

National Cancer Institute. 1994. *State Cancer Legislative Database Program.* Bethesda, MD: Division of Cancer Prevention and Control.

National Center for Health Statistics. 1977. *Development of the Design of the NCHS Hospital Discharge Survey.* Vital and health statistics, series 2, no. 39. Washington, D.C.: U.S. Government Printing Office.

National Committee for Quality Assurance. 1993. *Health Plan Employer Data and Information Set and User's Manual,* version 2.0. Washington, D.C.: National Committee for Quality Assurance.

National Committee for Quality Assurance. 1995. *HEDIS 2/5: Updated Specifications for HEDIS 2.0.* Washington, D.C.: National Committee for Quality Assurance.

National Research Council, Social Science Research Council, Committee on National Statistics, Commission on Behavioral and Social Sciences and Education. 1993. *Private Lives and Public Policies: Confidentiality and Accessibility of Government Statistics,* edited by G. T. Duncan, T. B. Jabine, and V. A. de Wolf. Washington, D.C.: National Academy Press.

Qualters, J. R., N. C. Lee, R. A. Smith, et al. 1992. Breast and cervical cancer surveillance, United States, 1973–1987. *Morb. Mortal. Wkly. Rep.,* 41:1–7.

Reis, L. A. G., B. F. Hankey, B. A. Miller, et al. 1991. *Cancer Statistics Review 1973–88.* Bethesda, MD: National Cancer Institute. NIH publication no. 91-2789.

Reynolds, G. H., D. L. McGee, and D. F. Stroup. 1989. Symposium on statistics in surveillance. *Stat. Med.,* 8:251–400.

Roos, N. P., C. D. Black, L. L. Roos, et al. 1995. A population-based approach to monitoring adverse outcomes of medical care. *Med. Care,* 33:127–138.

Siegel, P. Z., R. M. Brackbill, F. L. Frazier, et al. 1991. Behavioral risk factor surveillance, 1986–1990. *Morb. Mortal. Wkly. Rpt. CDC Surveill. Summ.,* 40:1–23.

Simonsen, L., M. Clark, D. F. Stroup, et al. 1997. The impact of influenza epidemics on mortality. *Am. J. Public Health* (in press).

Stroup, D. F., M. Wharton, K. Kafadar, et al. 1993. An evaluation of a method for detecting aberrations in public health surveillance data. *Am. J. Epidemiol.,* 137:373–380.

Terris, M. 1992. The Society for Epidemiologic Research (SER) and the future of epidemiology. *Am. J. Epidemiol.,* 136:909–915.

Teutsch, S. M., W. H. Herman, D. M. Dwyer, et al. 1984. Mortality among diabetic patients using continuous subcutaneous insulin-infusion pumps. *N. Engl. J. Med.,* 310:361–368.

Thacker, S. B. 1991. A war room for health. In: *Imminent Peril: Public Health in a Declining Economy,* edited by K. M. Cahill. New York: Twentieth Century Fund Press, pp. 97–103.

Thacker, S. B. 1992. The principles and practice of public health surveillance: use of data in public health practice. *Sante Publique* 4:43–49.

Thacker, S. B., and R. L. Berkelman. 1988. Public health surveillance in the United States. *Epidemiol. Rev.*, 10:164–190.

Thacker, S. B., and R. L. Berkelman. 1992. History of public health surveillance. In: *Public Health Surveillance*, edited by W. E. Halperin, E. L. Baker., and R. R. Monson. New York: Van Nostrand Reinhold.

Thacker, S. B., and D. F. Stroup. 1994. Future directions in public health surveillance. *Am. J. Epidemiol.*, 140:383–397.

Thacker, S. B., R. L. Berkelman, and D. F. Stroup. 1989. The science of public health surveillance. *J. Public Health Policy*, 10:187–203.

Van Grevenhof, P., C. G. Chute, and D. J. Ballard. 1991. A common and clonable environment to support research using patient data. Assessing the value of medical informatics. In: *Proceedings, Fifteenth Annual Symposium on Computer Applications in Medical Care*. Washington, D.C.

Whittle, J., E. P. Steinberg, G. F. Anderson, et al. 1991. Accuracy of Medicare claims data for estimation of cancer incidence and resection rates among elderly Americans. *Med. Care*, 29:1226–1236.

Williamson, G. D., J. T. Massey, H. B. Shulman, W. K. Sieber, and S. J. Smith. 1994. Symposium on quantitative methods for the utilization of multi-source data in public health. *Stat Med.*, 14(5/6/7).

CHAPTER 6

General Population Studies

WILLIAM W. EATON

Epidemiology is the study of diseases in populations, and services research in the context of epidemiology focuses on populations as well. A population is a group sharing a characteristic such as gender, occupation, workplace, race, nationality, age, and so forth. The general population is not limited to any particular class or characteristic but includes all persons without regard to special features. In the context of research studies, the ''general population'' usually refers to the individuals who normally reside in the locality of the study. Many epidemiologic studies involve large populations, such as a nation, a state, or even a county of several hundred thousand inhabitants. In such large studies, the general population includes individuals with a wide range of social and biologic characteristics, and this variation is helpful in generalizing the results. In the broadest sense, the ''general population'' refers to the human species.

The *natural history* is the onset, course, and outcome of a disease in its ''natural'' circumstances, i.e., without human intervention. The definition of ''natural'' sometimes leads to argument since the definition of ''human intervention,'' especially in the context of widespread public health and curative efforts for disease, can be unduly limiting in scope. Natural history thus excludes studies of specific clinical or preventive trials but includes observational studies of populations in the context of normal public health and medical systems. Follow-up studies of general populations—also the topic of this chapter—have the potential to provide the most valid data on the natural history of a disease.

This chapter considers the contributions of the population-based approach, including follow-up studies in the community, for health services research. The focus is on neither the disease in the general population nor the natural history of the disease; rather, it is on health services research set in this epidemiologic context. While the general population survey provides estimates of such epidemiologic parameters as prevalence of disease, the focus here is on the related parameters of need for service and demand. Focusing on the natural history of a disease is important for epidemiology generally, but in this chapter the focus is on the history of treatment, including failure to seek treatment.

The important potentials of the general population approach to health services research are in the study of the following:

1. Need for medical care
2. Demand for care and unmet need
3. Help seeking and barriers to care
4. Comorbidity, Berkson's bias, and use of health services
5. Relation of natural history of disease to the use of health services
6. Estimating the total cost of disease

The chapter presents examples of three studies: the National Institute of Mental Health (NIMH) Epidemiologic Catchment Area (ECA) Program, the Longitudinal Study on Aging (LSOA), and the Oxford Record Linkage Study (ORLS). These studies were chosen from among many possibilities to represent the entire life course, from birth to death; to include more than one national population; to span the range of medical problems from physical to psychiatric; and to exemplify and illustrate important potentials and limitations of general population follow-up studies in the community, for health services research. After finishing the chapter the reader should be able to evaluate the degree to which any given individual general population follow-up study has attained the potentials of the method and the degree to which it has successfully addressed the problems and limitations of the method.

Examples of Three Studies

The ECA Program

The NIMH sponsored the ECA Program from 1978 through 1985 as a response to the President's Commission on Mental Health, which recommended immediate efforts to gather reliable data on the incidence of mental health problems and the utilization of mental health services (President's Commission on Mental Health, 1978). The broad aims of the ECA Program were "to estimate the incidence and prevalence of mental disorders, to search for etiological clues, and to aid in the planning of health care facilities" (Eaton et al., 1981). The program involved sample surveys of populations living in the catchment areas of designated community mental health centers. The surveys were coordinated by the NIMH staff through a cooperative agreement funding mechanism and carried out by researchers at five universities: Yale University, in New Haven, Connecticut; the Johns Hopkins University, in Baltimore, Maryland; Washington University, in

St. Louis, Missouri; Duke University, in Durham, North Carolina; and the University of California, in Los Angeles, California. The broad goals of the ECA Program are described by Eaton et al. (1981) and Regier et al. (1984). The methods are described by Eaton et al. (1984) and Eaton and Kessler (1985). The cross-sectional results are described by Robins and Regier (1991) and in some 500 scientific papers published to date. A 10-year evaluation of the program reflects on its accomplishments and shortcomings (Eaton, 1994; Regier, 1994; Kessler, 1994; Shrout, 1994).

The ECA Program design included samples of about 3,500 in each of the five sites, ultimately yielding a pooled sample of 20,861. The measurement included a baseline face-to-face interview in the household, followed by brief telephone interviews after 3, 6, and 9 months and a follow-up personal interview after 1 year. At the Yale site, there was a 9-year follow-up for mortality (Bruce et al., 1994); at the St. Louis site, a follow-up after 12 years of part of the original sample is currently under way; and at the Baltimore site, a follow-up of the entire cohort of 3,481 household respondents is currently completing the field work phase.

Health services research was an integral part of the ECA Program from its inception. The core instruments used at all five sites included the NIMH Diagnostic Interview Schedule (DIS) (Robins et al., 1981), which obtained detailed symptomatic information on a broad range of specific psychiatric disorders. The core instrument also included a series of questions on the use of health services, including inpatient and outpatient services, in both the general medical sector and the specialty psychiatric sector (Shapiro et al., 1985). Health services research analyses were included in the initial presentation of results (Shapiro et al., 1984).

The LSOA

The LSOA is a collaborative effort of the U.S. National Center for Health Statistics (NCHS) and the National Institute on Aging (NIA). The NCHS conducts the Health Interview Survey (HIS) as part of its ongoing effort to describe the health status of the U.S. population (The National Health Interview Survey, 1985). The HIS involves a representative sample of the U.S. population interviewed in the household by permanent staff of the NCHS and the Bureau of the Census, with a basic set of questions on sociodemographic variables, disabilities, visits to the doctor, health conditions, and hospitalizations. In 1 year the HIS sample comprises about 100,000 individuals.

Supplements to the HIS are sometimes funded by other government agencies. In 1984 the NIA funded the Supplement on Aging (SOA) to the HIS for the following purposes:

1. To characterize the health and social status of people aged 55 years and over in the United States
2. To provide information about how psychosocial and environmental factors interact with health factors to influence the aging individual in a changing society
3. To provide a knowledge base for investigating issues of prevention and postponement of disability and dependency
4. To form the basis for a prospective study, the LSOA (Fitti and Kovar, 1987)

The sample for the SOA consisted of one-half of those in the 1984 HIS sample in the age range 55–64 year (yielding 4,651 completed interviews) and all those in the 1984 HIS sample who were 65 years of age and older (yielding 11,497 completed interviews), for a total sample of 16,148 (Fitti and Kovar, 1987). Questions for the SOA interview were drawn from many sources and pretested twice. The questionnaire supplement added about 1 h to the 30 min HIS basic questionnaire, containing information on family structure, community and social support, occupation and retirement, health conditions, measures of functioning, and aspects of nursing home stays.

The follow-up phase of the SOA became the LSOA (Fig. 6-1). The LSOA

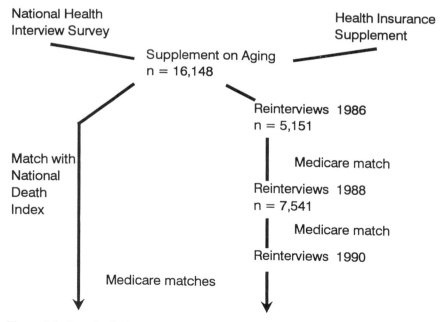

Figure 6-1. Longitudinal Study on Aging, redrawn from Kovar, Fitti, and Chyba, 1992.

includes matching of the SOA sample with the National Death Index for the years 1984–1990, matching of SOA sample individuals over the age of 65 years with Medicare files, and mail and telephone follow-ups of a selected sample of 7,527 SOA respondents who were 70 years and older in 1984 (Kovar et al., 1992). These follow-ups took place in 1986 (5,151 respondents only), 1988, and 1990. The LSOA has been used extensively in studying health services use by the elderly (e.g., Wolinsky and Johnson, 1991).

The ORLS

The ORLS was set up in 1962 to "follow the medical record of individuals from cradle to grave" (Acheson et al., 1961; Acheson, 1967; Baldwin et al., 1987). The following objectives were outlined by Acheson (1987):

1. To study the feasibility and cost of accumulating records of health events and linking them to personal and family files
2. To develop computer methods of record linkage
3. To study applications of these files in medical and operational research
4. To promote (if successful) the extension of the method to the national level

The study began with the population of 350,000 residents of Oxford County and was later expanded to a larger geographic area of about 2,000,000. The data consisted of abstracts of birth, death, and hospital admissions. At a later stage, data on psychiatric day patients and outpatients were added.

The ORLS is not a typical community study because no house-to-house survey was conducted. It is an example of a record-based approach to health services research, but the ORLS has a clearly defined population base, as well as systematic follow-up, which fits within the purview of this chapter. The ORLS is a *disease register,* which is defined here as a system of standardized record keeping for a general population in which records are linked over time and across health facilities. The ORLS is included as an exemplar of disease registers because it provides an informative contrast to the ECA and LSOA studies and because it has pioneered many efforts at record linkage that are sometimes crucial to follow-up of rare diseases. Other excellent examples of registers exist, often linked to specific diseases, such as the Danish Psychiatric Case Register (Dupont, 1983). The technology for record linkage and data storage has made large advances, and the potential for these studies is growing (Mortensen, 1995). In the future, record linkage systems are likely to be used more widely, for both etiologic studies and health services research.

Methodologic issues

Important methodologic issues of the general population approach and problems that must be addressed by researchers conducting such studies include the following:

1. Definition of the target population
2. Determination of sample size
3. Standardization of data
4. Response rate
5. Attrition

Definition of the target population. The best way to define the target population is not always clear, and different definitions have implications for the ultimate value of the results, as well as the feasibility of the study. The purest definition of a target population is a birth cohort of an entire nation, such as the British Perinatal Study, which included all births in Britain during a single week in March 1958 (Butler and Alberman, 1969). Other studies usually involve compromises of one form or another. The goal of the sampling procedure is that each respondent is selected into the sample with a known, and non-zero, probability. Strict probabilistic sampling characterizes high-quality epidemiologic surveys and is a requirement for generalization to the target population.

Most surveys are of the household-residing, noninstitutionalized population, where the survey technology for sampling and interviewing individuals is strongest (e.g., Sudman, 1976). The LSOA sample was drawn from the HIS, which is of the noninstitutionalized population, even though an important part of the focus population, the elderly, resides in nursing homes. Thus, nursing home residents were omitted even from the target population. The ECA design defined the target population as ''normal'' residents of previously established catchment areas. Sampling was conducted in two strata. The household-residing population was sampled via area probability methods or household listings provided by utility companies (e.g., Sudman, 1976). This stratum included short-stay group quarters, such as jails, hospitals, and dormitories. After making a list of the residents in each household, the interviewer asked the person answering the door whether there were any other individuals who ''normally'' resided there but were temporarily absent. ''Normally'' was defined as the presence of a bed reserved for the individual at the time of the interview. Temporarily absent residents were added to the household roster before the single respondent was chosen randomly. If a selected individual was temporarily absent, the interviewer made an appointment for a time after that person's return or conducted the interview at his or her temporary group quarters residence (i.e., in the hospital, jail, dormitory, or other place). The ECA sampled the institutional populations separately, by listing all institutions in the catchment area, as well as all nearby institutions that admitted residents of the catchment area. Then, the inhabitants of each institution were rostered and selected probabilistically. Sampling the institutional population required many more resources per sampled individual than the household sample because each institution had to be approached individually. Inclusion of temporary and long-stay group quarters is important for health services research because many of the group quarters are involved in provision of health services and because residents of group quarters may be high utilizers. The ultimate result of these procedures in the ECA was that each normal resident of the catchment area was sampled with a known probability.

The data base of the ORLS consists of births, deaths, and hospital admissions, which is a strong limitation. However, because of the catchmenting aspect of the British National Health Service, the data are not limited to a household-residing population, as is the LSOA.

It is not enough to crisply define a geographic area because different areas involve different limitations on the generalizability of results. A nationally representative sample, such as the LSOA, may seem to be the best. However, how does one apply the results of the national sample to a given local area, where decisions about services are made? In the ECA, the decision was made to select five separate sites of research to provide for replication of results across sites and to better understand the effects of local variation (Eaton et al., 1981). The ECA target population thus consisted, not of the nation, but rather of an awkward aggregation of catchment areas. Nevertheless, the ECA data were considered as benchmarks for a generation of research (Eaton, 1994) because there was sufficient variation in important sociodemographic variables to allow generalization to other large populations, that is, sufficiently large subgroups of young and old, men and women, married and unmarried, rich and poor, and so forth. Generalization to other target populations, such as Asian Americans or Native Americans, or to rural areas was not logical from the ECA. Note, however, that generalization from a national random sample to all rural areas or to small ethnic groups likewise would not always be possible. The point is that the target population should be chosen with a view toward later generalization.

Sample size. General population surveys are not efficient designs for rare disorders or unusual patterns of service use. Even for research on outcomes that are not rare, sample sizes are often larger than 1,000. A common statistic to be estimated in health services research is the proportion, for example, the proportion of the population visiting a health care provider. For a proportion, the precision is affected by the square root of the sample size (Blalock, 1979). If the distribution of the proportion is favorable—for example, between 30% and 70%—then a sample size of 1,000 produces precision that may be good enough for common sample surveys, such as for voter preference. For example, a proportion of 0.50 has a 95% confidence interval of 0.47–0.53 with a sample of 1,000. For rarer disorders or lower proportions of the sample using services, the confidence interval grows relative to the size of the proportion (i.e., 0.82–0.118 for a proportion of 0.10 and 0.004–0.160 for a proportion of 0.01). Often, there is interest in patterns of service use broken down by subpopulations, thus challenging the utility of samples with as few as 1,000 individuals. Each of the two case examples of community surveys (ECA and LSOA) has baseline samples in excess of 3,000, while the ORLS can undertake studies of rarer disorders with a much larger population base. It is important to estimate the precision of the sample for parameters of interest and the power of the sample to test the hypotheses of interest before beginning data collection.

Standardization of data collection. Assessment in epidemiology ideally should be undertaken with standardized measurement instruments that have known and acceptable reliability and validity. In community surveys and automated record systems, reliable and valid measurement must take place efficiently and under "field conditions." The amount of training for interviewers in household studies depends on the nature of the study. LSOA interviewers received about 1.5 days of training (Fitti and Kovar, 1987), while ECA interviewers received slightly more than 1 week (Munson et al., 1985). Telephone interviews, such as in the LSOA, can be systematically monitored by recording or listening in on a random basis (as long as the subject is made aware of this possibility), but it is difficult to monitor household interviews since it cannot be predicted exactly when and where the interview will take place. In automated data collection systems such as the ORLS, recording is often done under the auspices of the medical record systems, with data such as the diagnosis recorded by the physician. It cannot be presumed that the physician's diagnosis is "standardized" and therefore more reliable than other interview or record data. In fact, there is significant variation in diagnosis among physicians. Research using measurements and diagnoses recorded by the physician—as in record linkage systems such as the ORLS—ideally should include studies of reliability and validity (e.g., Loffler et al., 1994).

The ECA Program involved a somewhat innovative interview, the DIS (Robins et al., 1981). The DIS was designed to resemble a typical psychiatric interview, in which the questions are highly dependent on answers already given. For example, if an individual responds positively to a question about the occurrence of panic attacks, a series of questions about that particular response are asked; if the response to the question on panic is negative, the interviewer skips to the next section. In effect, the interview adapts to the responses of the subject so that more questions are asked where more information is needed. The high degree of structure in the DIS required more than 1 week of training, as well as attention to the visual properties of the interview booklet itself. The result was that the interviewer could follow instructions regarding the flow of the interview and the recording of data smoothly so as not to offend or alienate the respondent. Household survey questionnaires are becoming increasingly adaptive and response-dependent because more information can be provided in a shorter amount of time with adaptive interviews. Inexpensive laptop computers will facilitate such adaptive interviewing. Self-administered, computerized admission procedures are becoming more widely disseminated in the health care system, expanding the data base and facilitating the retrieval and linkage of records.

The reliability and validity of measurement are usually assessed prior to beginning a field study. Usually, the assessment involves pilot tests on samples of convenience to determine the optimal order of the questions, the time required for each section, and whether any questions are unclear or offensive. Debriefing subjects in these pilot tests is often helpful. The next step is a test of reliability and validity. Many pretests select samples from populations according to their health or services use characteristics in order to generate enough variation in responses to adequately estimate reliability and validity. To economize, such pretests are often conducted in clinical settings. However, such pretests do not predict reliability and validity under the field conditions of household interviews. The ECA Program design involved reliability and validity assessment in a hospital setting (Robins et al., 1981) and later under field conditions (Anthony et al., 1985; Helzer et al., 1985). The reliability and validity of the DIS were lower in the household setting.

Response and nonresponse. The rate of response is a critical feature of any research study, but it is sometimes more difficult to achieve an acceptable response rate in community surveys as compared with research in medical settings. High-quality surveys are strictly probabilistic in that respondents are designated independently through a randomization process and substitutions are not permitted. The *response rate* is the proportion of those designated who actually complete an interview.

In a field survey, the interviewer is a guest in the respondent's household and can be asked to leave at any time. The explanation of the purpose of the interview, the logic for selecting that particular subject, the credibility of the materials that identify the interviewers as bonafide, and the procedures for guaranteeing anonymity or confidentiality may require more forceful or clear justification than in a medical setting, where the environment is more predictable and supportive of the data collection effort. It rarely occurs that an interview is terminated by the respondent once it has started (e.g., less than 1% in the LSOA or the ECA); what is more important is the failure to begin an interview.

Nonresponse can bias the results because hard-to-reach respondents, or those who refuse to participate, can be different in their health and health services characteristics from those who participate (Von Korff et al., 1985; Cottler et al., 1987). Regularly scheduled household health surveys conducted by the U.S. Government, such as the SOA, typically achieve a response rate above 90% (SOA rate of 96.7% reported by Fitti and Kovar, 1987). Private organizations involved in health surveys typically report response rates of 70–80%. (The response rate in the ECA Program baseline varied from less than 70% in Los Angeles to above 80% in St. Louis [Leaf et al., 1991].) Special incentive procedures may be used to obtain participation by hard-to-reach or reluctant respondents, and nonresponse weights can be developed to adjust for nonresponse bias (Kessler et al., 1995).

Sample attrition. *Sample attrition* is the decline in participation in the study after the initial response. Sample attrition takes the form of (1) mortality, (2) loss of contact with the individual, and (3) refusal to participate further in the study. Sample attrition in follow-up studies is analogous to non-response in cross-sectional surveys, as described above. However, this occurs often because of the passage of time and the increment of response burden, and it is more complex because of the dynamic interplay of health- and service-related events of the respondent with study participation. Attrition can lead to bias in study results because data on outcomes in later stages of the follow-up are not available for a subsample.

Mortality is a source of attrition that is directly related to health status and to age. In the ECA study, older age, major depressive disorder, and cognitive impairment all predicted mortality in follow-up years (Bruce et al., 1994; Liu and Anthony, 1989; Kouzis et al., 1995). A variety of health-related statuses predicted mortality in the LSOA (Steinbach, 1992; Rakowski, 1992). Mortality is a crucially important outcome for epidemiologic studies in general. For health services research, an implication of mortality is that the record of health services use for an individual, in the period during which usage is likely to be high, may be unavailable because the respondent has died and cannot supply the information or provide the authorization for searching records, which then must be obtained from the next of kin.

Refusal and loss of contact are other sources of attrition. Additional refusals after the first baseline participation may occur because the cumulative burden of response has risen above a threshold set by the respondent due to an intervening event, whether health-related or not. Studies of attrition in the ECA surveys after 1 year (Eaton et al., 1992) and after 14 years (Badawi et al., 1996) do not reveal important biases among refusers. In contrast, people with certain types of health and mental health problems are much more likely to be lost to follow-up

(Eaton et al., 1992; Badawi et al., 1996). In the ECA, about 24% had died after 14 years (Table 6-1), about 12% of those presumed to be alive were not located, and another 9% did not agree to continue participating. The 73% of survivors who completed interviews amounted to about 50% of the individuals originally designated as respondents in 1981. In the LSOA, higher mortality but slightly fewer refusals and failures to locate occurred (Table 6-1).

Nonresponse and attrition are different in record linkage systems. The definition of the health event is certainly more circumscribed, and its relation to clinical disease is uncertain. However, once that factor is accounted for, nonresponse and even long-term attrition are likely to be so small as to be trivial. Consider the example of schizophrenia. In a population-based survey of schizophrenia, it might be necessary to interview or examine 5,000 or more persons to generate a sample of only 50 schizophrenics. If the response rate were 80%, there might be only 4,000 individuals successfully interviewed and only 40 schizophrenics. Studies have shown that about 80% of schizophrenics eventually see a psychiatrist over their lifetime and would be entered into a comprehensive psychiatric case register (Eaton, 1985). There is little or no record loss once the individual has entered the facility, so the same 40 schizophrenics might be in the record-based research study as in the field study. The record linkage system in Denmark

Table 6-1. Attrition in the Longitudinal Study on Aging (LSOA), for the period 1984–1990, and the Baltimore Epidemiologic Catchment Area (ECA-B) 1981–1993/4

	LSOA		ECA-B	
	Frequency	*Percent*	*Frequency*	*Percent*
Baseline completion[a]		96.4%		94.9%
Complete	4,141	55.0%	1,920	55.2%
Refusal[b]	430	5.7%	298	8.6%
Not located[c]	701	9.3%	415	11.9%
Total Survivors	5,272	70.0%	2,633	75.6%
Deceased[d]	2,255	30.0%	848	24.4%
Total deceased and survivors	7,527	100.0%	3,481	100.0%
Complete/survivors		78.5%		72.9%

[a]This figure is the percentage of households selected in which a respondent was actually designated.

[b]The LSOA is a telephone follow-up in which informants' telephone reports are included as complete interviews.

[c]In the LSOA, "not located" includes those in institutions and/or mentally or physically incapable of responding (12% of total "not located"); in the ECA "not located" includes all persons whose address could not be verified by phone or interview contact.

[d]The deceased do not include the most recent files of the National Death Index (1990 for the LSOA, 1995 for the ECA-B).

Sources: LSOA: Kovar et al. (1992), Table H and Fig. 4; ECA-B: Badawi et al. (1996), Table 1 and Fig. 1.

has the advantage of covering a much larger population (e.g., the population of 5,000,000 persons in the nation of Denmark). The diagnostic ability of the psychiatrist regarding this particular disorder is likely to be much higher than that of the interviewer in the field survey. This logic leads to the conclusion that, for schizophrenia, case registers are more cost-effective sources of information than household-oriented field studies. This logic pertains even more strongly to diseases that are so impairing that they inevitably lead to hospitalization, such as leukemia, cystic fibrosis, multiple sclerosis, and so forth. The point of this discussion is to show that there is no advantage of the household vs. record-based method that pertains across the range of illnesses.

Potentials of the Community-Based Approach

Need for medical care

The community-based approach potentially produces the best assessment of need for services in a population. No other approach has this capability. The record-based method, such as the ORLS, suffers in comparison because it can be used to obtain estimates only of demand for services but not of the need for them.

The definition and measurement of need are problematic. The definition of need necessarily depends on the availability and effectiveness of services. An individual can have an incurable or debilitating condition, but if no effective treatment is available, it may not be useful to define that individual as in need of health care. Likewise, all individuals suffer through health problems at one time or another. In the general population, the prevalence of any illness is very high (Antonovsky, 1979). If all problems are defined as potentially deserving of health care, there is no imaginable health care system that could respond. Therefore, a threshold of need must be established, and this threshold will incorporate the ability of the health care system to respond to need.

Measurement of need can be through a variety of approaches. One approach is to diagnose diseases and conditions and to relate their presence systematically to need. The problems with this approach are that not all diseases and conditions need treatment and that there is large variation in the severity of disorders and conditions in terms of their need for services.

Measures of distress and demoralization help address the issue of need. Distress is necessarily subjective, but there are a variety of reliable scales with good validity, such as the General Health Questionnaire (Goldberg, 1972), the Perceived Stress Scale (Cohen et al., 1983), the Psychiatric Epidemiology Research Interview (PERI) Demoralization Scale (Dohrenwend et al., 1980), and others (reviewed in McDowell and Newell, 1987). Health conditions are associated with distress, and their treatment relieves distress. A problem in measurement is that the distress is sometimes measured generally, not related to any specific disease; therefore, the specific type of treatment needed may not be obvious.

Measures of functioning also help to address the issue of need for service. *Functioning* is the ability to perform certain activities or behaviors. Impairment due to a disease or condition is revealed in lowered functioning, and treatment improves functioning. Popular measures of functioning include the activities of daily living (ADL) scales (McDowell and Newell, 1987), used in the LSOA as well as at several sites of the ECA Program. As with measures of distress and demoralization, the functioning scales are usually general, making it difficult to specify in detail the type of need.

A possible error in the design of the ECA surveys was too much reliance on diagnosis as a measure of need. One ECA analysis combined measures of distress with diagnostic measures to obtain a more balanced measure of need (Shapiro et al., 1986). Nevertheless, even in that analysis, omission of variables related to functioning remained a limitation to the needs assessment.

Population-based measures of need can be used to design the health care system. For example, Kramer (1995) has estimated the need for psychiatrists in the United States as a whole, using needs assessment data from the ECA Program.

Demand and unmet need

Demand is the population expression of request for health care services. Many individuals below a threshold of need nevertheless request services (inappropriate demand); many individuals with a need for service do not request it (unmet need). Inappropriate demand is an important nuisance, leading to waste in the distribution of health care resources. Unmet need may lead to complications, comorbidities, impairments, and death. Only where need is measured in a community population can inappropriate demand and unmet need be studied: studies with samples from treatment populations obviously do not involve individuals with unmet need, and studies based in one treatment agency or at one point in time will miss many health care visits that together may constitute inappropriate demand.

A popular model of the use of health care services in the population is the Andersen-Aday P-E-N model (Andersen, 1968, 1995; Aday and Andersen, 1974). The P-E-N model categorizes predictors of health care utilization, that is, demand for services, into the three classes of predisposing features (P), enabling features (E), and aspects of need (N). Predisposing features include sociodemographic variables, such as age and gender; social structural factors, such as socioeconomic position and education; certain beliefs about health; and factors related to the physical environment. Enabling resources exist at the level of the community, such as the availability of health facilities, and at the level of the individual, such as the means and know-how to get to health facilities and the ability to pay for health care. Need is the biologic imperative of disease, as evaluated by the professional, and the pain or symptom as experienced by the individual. Analyses of the LSOA have been designed around the P-E-N model. For example, Wolinsky and Johnson (1991) are able to predict as much as 25% of the variance in health services utilization by aged persons, using regression models including measures of predisposing, enabling, and need factors.

A large amount of unmet need is a flag that the health service system is not working properly and may lead to the design and provision of public information and outreach services. For example, analyses of the ECA Program data revealed that about 50% of those meeting diagnostic criteria for major depressive disorder had not seen a professional for treatment within the prior 6 months (Shapiro et al., 1984). Since there exist well-established treatments for depression, the NIMH began a public awareness program, called Depression/Awareness, Recognition, and Treatment (D/ART), to lower the amount of unmet need in the population (Regier et al., 1988).

If there exist particular types of population with a high degree of unmet need, such as groups defined by gender, race, or socioeconomic status, the unmet need is unbalanced and there is presumably inequity in the distribution of services. In terms of the P-E-N model, there is relatively equitable access to care when sociodemographic characteristics and need predict utilization but inequitable access when use of health services is better predicted by social structure, health beliefs, and enabling resources (Andersen, 1995).

Equity of access to care also can be studied in record linkage systems but only after the individual has entered the system. For example, referral to highly specialized care may differ between different regions or different hospitals. In the Oxford region, there was concern that persons under 55 years with stroke who were admitted to nonteaching hospitals might not be investigated thoroughly for conditions, such as an aneurysm, which are amenable to surgery. In fact, data from individual hospitals showed that those admitted to nonteaching hospitals had much lower rates of surgery than those admitted to teaching hospitals. Record linkage, however, permitted taking account of transfers, showing that about 25% of those admitted to nonteaching hospitals, and the same percentage admitted to teaching hospitals, eventually were diagnosed with an aneurysm and that about 13% of both sets of admissions underwent surgery (Goldacre, 1987).

Help seeking and illness behavior

A central advantage of community surveys is that processes leading to the use, and the avoidance, of services can be studied. This involves a study of factors that influence unmet need and inappropriate demand. *Illness behavior* is the way persons respond to bodily indications which they experience as abnormal. . . . [It] involves the manner in which persons monitor their bodies, define and interpret their symptoms, take remedial actions, and utilize the health-care system. (Mechanic, 1983, p. 591)

The process by which persons seek help is complicated, and there are typically large differences between populations with the same physical problems. Mechanic (1978) lists a range of determinants that affect the response to bodily deviations: perceived salience, perceived seriousness, extent of disruption of activities, frequency and persistence, tolerance thresholds, knowledge and cultural assumptions, need for denial, competing needs, alternative interpretations, and accessibility of treatment. None of these factors is strictly determined by the bodily process or deviation itself. Each of these determinants may differ widely among subgroups of the population and strongly affects the use of services (Leaf et al., 1986, 1987, 1988). The challenge for the health services researcher conducting a community survey is to include sufficient detail on these processes to develop a compelling explanatory model for predicting services use. The community survey is the most common method for studying illness behavior, though it is not without its weaknesses (Mechanic, 1983). The efficiency of the assessment procedures that is required in epidemiologic surveys and the breadth of help-seeking determinants, as described above, may lead to omission of crucial illness variables that hinder clear interpretation of the data, especially regarding the relative influence of help-seeking factors vs. illness factors per se.

Inappropriate demand is an important characteristic of the efficiency of the service system. It is possible to identify individual dramatic instances of inappropriate demand, such as cases of malingering or Munchhausen's syndrome, in the context of a given treatment setting. However, the volume of inappropriate demand can be approximated only in a community survey with a longitudinal component. This volume is likely to be affected in only a small degree by dramatic instances such as Munchhausen's syndrome; rather, it is more likely to be affected by variations in help-seeking behaviors as listed above. For example, in the ECA Program, it was shown that the psychiatric disorder with the most immediate and strongest linkage to treatment seeking was panic disorder; but in many cases, individuals sought treatment in the general health care system, where they are likely to receive expensive, and possibly inappropriate, diagnostic tests related to cardiovascular problems (Boyd, 1986).

Comorbidity, Berkson's bias, and use of the health service system

The existence of more than one illness in the same individual has important effects on the use of the health care system. *Berkson's bias* is the tendency for individuals in the community with more than one symptom or disorder to seek treatment at a higher rate than those with just one symptom or disorder (Lilienfeld and Stolley, 1994). As a result, cases defined by disease status or some aspect of their services use are more likely to have comorbidity with other disorders than are cases which might be identified through a population-based survey. This leads to problems in interpretation of results because the relation of an exposure to the comorbid disorder, or treatment for it, may be misinterpreted as being the result of a relation to the disorder that is the focus of the study. When community studies collect data on many disorders, they can study this phenomenon. For example, studies in the ECA showed that depressive symptoms were more likely to occur without panic in the psychiatric treatment system and with panic in the general health services system (Eaton and Chilcoat, 1992).

Comorbidities may be influenced by the health services system. Some comorbidity may be the result of complications of treatment, as well as unexpected side effects or long-term consequences. In some cases, comorbidity may be an artifact of treatment. For example, the ECA Follow-up Study revealed an increased risk for onset of type II diabetes among individuals who had, at baseline, met the criteria for diagnosis of major depressive disorder. However, it may have been the case that treatment for depression led to uncovering the diabetes, thus producing the finding (Eaton et al., 1996). As another example, linkage of records may reveal useful information on prodromal symptoms that can reduce onsets of disease. Hobbs et al. (1976), in a study from the ORLS, found that patients with colon cancer had been treated recently for diverticulitis in excess of the rate in the general population; likewise, patients with brain tumors had been treated recently for certain conditions of the central nervous system at higher rates than the general population. It would seem possible that the colon and brain cancers might have been present and detectable at the earlier visits for diverticulitis and central nervous system conditions, respectively. This information could lead to more effective early identification and treatment.

Natural history of disease and use of services

The longitudinal aspects of follow-up and linkage research allow considerable insight into services use that is not available in cross-sectional surveys or more general record-based approaches. Concepts for assessing the dynamics of natural history include lifetime, period, and point prevalence; first incidence and attack rate; and duration of episodes (Eaton, 1995). Any population-based follow-up study has the potential to define operationally and to measure these concepts, but the operational definitions and the accuracy of measurement differ between register-based and survey-based approaches. Table 6-2 shows the rough equivalence of the two approaches. The survey approach uses a question or series of questions with the phrasing shown. For example, for lifetime prevalence, ''Have you ever had a heart attack?'' might be the survey question. To determine lifetime

Table 6-2. Survey and register estimates of parameters of natural history

Parameter	Survey	Hospital Register
Point prevalence	"Are You . . ."	Current residents
Lifetime prevalence	"Have you ever . . ."	Any admission since birth
Period prevalence	"Since xx, have you . . ."	Residents + admissions during interval
Attack rate	Difference in point prevalence at two waves	Admissions during interval
First incidence	Difference in lifetime prevalence at two waves	First admissions
Duration	"How long . . ."	Length of stay

prevalence in the context of a case register requires complete records that are linked across time from birth forward and across all possible facilities—a difficult challenge. Except for the first incidence, a simple analogue, like the first admission rate, is used. Here, the more difficult problem is for the survey approach, which must determine lifetime prevalence at baseline to identify those at risk and then repeat the survey at least once sometime in the future to identify new cases among those at risk. These measures focus, potentially at least, on the need side (survey) and demand side (register). In the early stages of the National Health Survey, there were a series of studies assessing the accuracy of respondents' reports of health services use in field surveys by comparison with medical records (Yaffe et al., 1978). The results showed that a sizable proportion of survey respondents did not report medical events occurring more than a few weeks or months prior to the interview (depending on the severity of the event). Attempts to directly compare population estimates of demand from parallel surveys and record-based approaches are rare (Manderscheid et al., 1993).

Measures of the natural history of disease are related to health services research. First, they contribute to the prevalence of disorder, which produces demand on the services system (the age schedule of first incidence contributes to lifetime prevalence, as in Kramer et al. [1980]; the duration and attack rate produce the point prevalence, under certain conditions, as in Kramer [1957]). Second, all of these indicators are influenced by, and serve as indicators of, the relative performance of the services system. As such, the need for benchmark estimates of measures of natural history is paramount. For example, there are many studies of the course and outcome of episodic psychiatric disorders, like major depressive disorder (e.g., the collaborative study of depression [Keller et al., 1992]), and major efforts are under way to develop treatment guidelines for depression in the context of primary care (Depression Guidelines Panel, 1993). However, except for the Baltimore ECA Follow-up Study, there are no population-based estimates of the duration of the first or of recurrent episodes or

Table 6-3. Number of hospital episodes and people treated for selected diseases in the Oxford region, 1974–1978

Disease	Episodes	People
Multiple sclerosis	1,268	759
Hemophilia	1,184	316
Cystic fibrosis	182	96
Congenital hypothyroidism	9	9

Source: Adapted from Goldacre (1987), Table 18.8.

of the probability of recurrence. Estimates of these parameters of natural history originating from the treatment system are suspect because so many depressive episodes do not lead to treatment, and those that do may be unusual in terms of natural history.

The simple unduplication of records that occurs in a register system can be illuminating in understanding the need for services and in planning services around persons instead of episodes. The focus on natural history involves the notion of a career of services use, instead of episodes of care. Unduplication of serious chronic illnesses via the ORLS is displayed in Table 6-3. With data on episodes that are not linked, it is difficult to estimate the number of persons who will need care. Linking the data reveals the size of the problem in a more useful form. Likewise, consideration of natural history indicators in detail may reveal patterns of care not available in simple episode data. For example, Table 6-4 compares two geriatric hospitals in the Oxford region. Hospital A, somewhat larger, appears to have much shorter lengths of stay (average of 29 days vs. 120 days for hospital B). The difference in length of stay appears to arise from discharge and readmission of the same patients repeatedly, instead of fewer, longer admissions, as in hospital B. Differences such as these will become ever more complex as policies with stronger constraints on length of stay, readmission, and other indicators of natural history evolve.

Table 6-4. Durations per episode and per person in selected geriatric hospitals in the Oxford region

	Number of Available Beds/Year	Number of Discharges/Year	Length of Stay (Days)/Episode	Number of People Treated	Duration (Days) of Total Stay/Person
Hospital A	194	2,302	29	539	126
Hospital B	107	312	120	241	156

Source: Goldacre (1987), Tables 18.5 and 18.6.

Costs

The direct costs of health treatments can be measured with data from the treatment system. However, the total cost of ill health includes indirect costs due to mortality, decrements in functioning that lead to loss of income, and burden on others. The economic costs of disease are important in establishing priorities for research and treatment, and direct treatment costs do not always dominate the picture. For example, using ECA and other data, Rice et al. (1991) estimate that the total cost for 1985 associated with alcohol, drug use, and mental disorders amounted to $218 billion: $51 billion was associated with direct treatment and support, and the remaining costs, about three-quarters of the total, were associated with reduced productivity; foregone future productivity due to mortality; and costs associated with increases in crime and accidents due to alcohol, drug use, and mental disorders. Various studies of the LSOA show the predictive relation of symptoms (Boult et al., 1991), physical activity (Rakowski, 1992), and preventive programs such as mammography (Mor et al., 1992) to functioning, mortality, and costs. Longitudinal data form an important part of the cost picture (Wolinsky et al., 1994). Thus, community surveys provide data for a more complete picture of costs than is available through statistics from the treatment system.

Even though community surveys appear to have access to more complete cost data, they may be less accurate than data based on the service system itself for complex treatment costs. An individual patient may be able to report on functioning and social costs but not be aware of the direct costs of treatment since there are so many sources of payment. Also, the true direct cost of care may necessitate averaging over many patients.

Conclusion

The preeminent advantage of population-based studies for health services research is their ability to estimate the need for services. When coupled with estimates of demand for services, the study of access to care is possible. Studies of need and access are hard to accomplish in other research designs. When longitudinal follow-up is included, the information becomes much richer because need and access may be more clearly understood when considered in a longitudinal framework, inappropriate patterns of use may be more easily identified, and total costs can be estimated.

References

Acheson, E. D. 1967. *Medical Record Linkage*. London: Oxford University Press.
Acheson, E. D. 1987. Introduction. In: *Textbook of Medical Record Linkage*, edited by

J. A. Baldwin, E. D. Acheson, and W. J. Graham. Oxford: Oxford University Press, pp. 1–12.

Acheson, E. D., S. C. Truelove, and L. J. Witts. 1961. National epidemiology. *Br. Med. J.*, 1:668.

Aday, L. A., and R. M. Andersen. 1974. A framework for the study of access to medical care. *Health Serv. Res.*, 9:208–220.

Andersen, R. M. 1968. Behavioral model of families. Use of health services. In: *Research Series No. 25*. Chicago, IL: Center for Health Administration Studies, University of Chicago.

Andersen, R. M. 1995. Revisiting the behavioral model and access to medical care: does it matter? *J. Health Soc. Behav.*, 36:1–10.

Anthony, J. C., M. F. Folstein, A. Romanoski, et al. 1985. Comparison of the lay diagnostic interview schedule and a standardized psychiatric diagnosis: experience in eastern Baltimore. *Arch. Gen. Psychiatry*, 42:667–675.

Antonovsky, A. 1979. Studying health instead of disease. In: *Health, Stress, and Coping*. San Francisco: Jossey-Bass, pp. 12–37.

Badawi, M. A., W. W. Eaton, J. Myllyluoma, et al. 1996. Psychopathology and attrition in the Baltimore ECA follow-up 1981–1996. Unpublished.

Baldwin, J. A., E. D. Acheson, and J. W. Graham, eds. 1987. *Textbook of Medical Record Linkage*. Oxford: Oxford University Press.

Blalock, H. M. 1979. *Social Statistics*, 2nd ed. New York: McGraw-Hill.

Boult, C. J., P. Murphy, V. Sloane, et al. 1991. The relation of dizziness to functional decline. *J. Am. Geriatr. Soc.*, 39:858–861.

Boyd, J. H. 1986. Use of mental health services for the treatment of panic disorder. *Am. J. Psychiatry*, 143:1569–1574.

Bruce, M. L., P. J. Leaf, G. P. F. L. Rozal, et al. 1994. Psychiatric status and 9-year mortality data in the New Haven Epidemiologic Catchment Area Study. *Am. J. Psychiatry*, 151:716–721.

Butler, N. R., and E. D. Alberman. 1969. *Perinatal Problems: The Second Report of the 1958 British Perinatal Survey*. Edinburgh: E & S Livingston, Ltd.

Cohen, S. T., R. Kamarck, and J. Mermelstein. 1983. A global measure of perceived stress. *J. Health Soc. Behav.*, 24:385–396.

Cottler, L. B., J. F. Zipp, L. N. Robins, et al. 1987. Difficult-to-recruit respondents and their effect on prevalence estimates in an epidemiologic survey. *Am. J. Epidemiol.*, 125:329–339.

Depression Guidelines Panel. 1993. *Depression in Primary Care. Detection and Diagnosis*, vol. 1. Rockville, MD: Agency for Health Care Policy and Research.

Dohrenwend, B. P., P. E. Shrout, G. Egri, et al. 1980. Nonspecific psychological distress and other dimensions of psychopathology. *Arch. Gen. Psychiatry*, 37:1229–1236.

Dupont, A. 1983. A national psychiatric case register as tool for mental health planning, research, and administration. In: *Information Support to Mental Health Programs*, edited by E. Laska, W. H. Gulbinat, and D. A. Regier. New York: Human Sciences Press, pp. 257–274.

Eaton, W. W. 1985. Epidemiology of schizophrenia. *Epidemiol. Rev.*, 7:105–126.

Eaton, W. W. 1994. The NIMH Epidemiologic Catchment Area program: implementation and major findings. *Int. J. Methods Psychiatr. Res.*, 4:103–112.

Eaton, W. W. 1995. Studying the natural history of psychopathology. In: *Textbook in*

Psychiatric Epidemiology, edited by M. Tsuang, M. Tohen, and G. Zahner. New York: Wiley-Liss, pp. 157–177.

Eaton, W. W., H. K. Armenian, J. Gallo, et al. 1996. Depression and risk for onset of type II diabetes: a prospective, population-based study. *Diabetes Care* 19(10): 1097–1101.

Eaton, W. W., J. C. Anthony, S. Tepper, et al. 1992. Psychopathology and attrition in the Epidemiologic Catchment Area surveys. *Am. J. Epidemiol.,* 135:1051–1059.

Eaton, W. W., and H. Chilcoat. 1992. The latent structure of anxiety and depression in treated and untreated samples of two U.S. populations. In: *Primary Health Care and Psychiatric Epidemiology,* edited by B. Cooper, and R. Eastwood. London: Routledge, pp. 307–318.

Eaton, W. W., C. E. Holzer, M. R. Von Korff , et al. 1984. The design of the ECA surveys: the control and measurement of error. *Arch. Gen. Psychiatry,* 41:942–948.

Eaton, W. W., and L. G. Kessler, eds. 1985. *Epidemiologic Field Methods in Psychiatry: The NIMH Epidemiologic Catchment Area Program.* Orlando, FL: Academic Press.

Eaton, W. W., D. A. Regier, B. Z. Locke, et al. 1981. The Epidemiologic Catchment Area program of the National Institute of Mental Health. *Public Health Rep.,* 96:319–325.

Fitti, J. E., and M. G. Kovar. 1987. The supplement on aging to the 1984 National Health Interview Survey. *Vital Health Stat.,* 21:1–115.

Goldacre, M. J. 1987. Implications of record linkage for health services management. In: *Textbook of Medical Record Linkage,* edited by J. A. Baldwin, E. D. Acheson, and W. J. Graham. Oxford: Oxford University Press, pp. 305–317.

Goldberg, D. 1972. *The Detection of Psychiatric Illness by Questionnaire.* London: Oxford University Press.

Helzer, J. E., L. N. Robins, L. T. McEvoy, et al. 1985. A comparison of clinical and diagnostic interview schedule diagnoses: physician reexamination of lay-interviewed cases in the general population. *Arch. Gen. Psychiatry,* 42:657–666.

Hobbs, M. S. T., A. S. Fairbairn, E. D. Acheson, et al. 1976. The study of disease associations from linked records. *Br. J. Prev. Soc. Med.,* 141:30–44.

Keller, M. B., P. W. Lavori, T. I. Mueller, et al. 1992. Time to recovery, chronicity, and levels of psychopathology in major depression: a 5-year prospective follow-up of 431 subjects. *Arch. Gen. Psychiatry,* 49:809–816.

Kessler, R. C. 1994. Building on the ECA: the national comorbidity survey and the children's ECA. *Int. J. Methods Psychiatr. Res.,* 4:81–94.

Kessler, R. C., R. J. A. Little, and R. M. Groves. 1995. Advances in strategies for minimizing and adjusting for survey nonresponse. *Epidemiol. Rev.,* 17:192–204.

Kouzis, A., W. W. Eaton, and P. Leaf. 1995. Psychopathology and mortality in the general population. *Soc. Psychiatry Psychiatr. Epidemiol.,* 30:165–170.

Kovar, M. G., J. E. Fitti, and M. Chyba. 1992. *The Longitudinal Study of Aging: 1984–90.* Hyattsville, MD: U.S. Department of Health and Human Services.

Kramer, M. A. 1957. Discussion of the concepts of incidence and prevalence as related to epidemiologic studies of mental disorders. *Am. J. Public Health,* 47:826–840.

Kramer, M. 1995. Projected changes in the population of the United States—1990, 2000, and 2010: implications for mental health and primary care. *Int. J. Methods Psychiatr. Res.,* 5:123–137.

Kramer, M., M. Von Korff, and L. Kessler. 1980. The lifetime prevalence of mental disorders: estimation, uses, and limitations. *Psychol. Med.*, 10:429–435.

Leaf, P. J., M. L. Bruce, and G. L. Tischler. 1986. The differential effect of attitudes on the use of mental health services. *Soc. Psychiatry,* 21:187–192.

Leaf, P. J., M. L. Bruce, G. L. Tischler, et al. 1987. The relationship between demographic factors and attitudes toward mental health services. *J. Commun. Psychol.,* 15:275–284.

Leaf, P. J., M. L. Bruce, G. L. Tischler, et al. 1988. Factors affecting the utilization of speciality and general medical mental health services. *Med. Care,* 26:9–26.

Leaf, P. J., M. M. Livingston, G. L.Tischler, M. M. Weissman, et al. 1985. Contact with health professionals for the treatment of psychiatric and emotional problems. *Med. Care,* 23:1322–1337.

Leaf, P. J., J. K. Myers, and L. T. McEvoy. 1991. Procedures used in the Epidemiologic Catchment Area Study. In: *Psychiatric Disorders in America,* edited by L. N. Robins, and D. A. Regier. New York: The Free Press, pp. 11–32.

Lilienfeld, D. E., and P. D. Stolley. 1994. *Foundations of Epidemiology.* New York: Oxford University Press.

Liu, I., and J. C. Anthony. 1989. Using the ''Mini-Mental State'' Examination to predict elderly subjects' completion of a follow-up interview. *Am. J. Epidemiol.,* 130:416–422.

Loffler, W., H. Hafner, B. Fatkenheuer, et al. 1994. Validation of Danish case register diagnosis for schizophrenia. *Acta Pschiatr. Scand.,* 90:196–203.

Manderscheid, R. W., D. S. Rae, W. E. Narrow, et al. 1993. Congruence of service utilization estimates from the Epidemiologic Catchment Area project and other sources. *Arch Gen Psychiatry,* 50:108–114.

McDowell, J., and C. Newell. 1987. *Measuring Health: A Guide to Rating Scales and Questionnaires.* New York: Oxford University Press.

Mechanic, D. 1978. *Medical Sociology,* 2nd ed. New York: The Free Press.

Mechanic, D. 1983. The experience and expression of distress: the study of illness behavior and medical utilization. In: *Handbook of Health, Health Care, and the Health Professions,* edited by D. Mechanic. New York: The Free Press, pp. 591–607.

Mor, V., J. T. Pacala, and W. Rakowski. 1992. Mammography for older women: Who uses, who benefits? *J. Gerontol.,* 47:43–49.

Mortensen, P. B. 1995. The untapped potential of case registers and record-linkage studies in psychiatric epidemiology. *Epidemiol. Rev.,* 17:205–209.

Munson, M. L., H. Orvaschel, E. A. Skinner, et al. 1985. Interviewers: characteristics, training and field work. In: *Epidemiologic Field Methods in Psychiatry: The NIMH Epidemiologic Catchment Area Program,* edited by W. W. Eaton, and L. G. Kessler. Orlando, FL: Academic Press, pp. 69–83.

The National Health Interview Survey design, 1973–1984, and procedures, 1975–1983, *Vital Health Statistics,* 1985, series 1, number 18.

President's Commission on Mental Health. 1978. *Report to the President from the President's Commission on Mental Health.* Washington, D.C.: U.S. Government Printing Office.

Rakowski, W. V. M. 1992. The association of physical activity with mortality among older adults in the Longitudinal Study of Aging (1984–1988). *J. Gerontol. Med. Sci.,* 47:M122–M129.

Regier, D. A. 1994. ECA contributions to national policy and further research. *Int. J. Methods Psychiatr. Res.,* 4:73–80.

Regier, D. A., R. M. A. Hirschfeld, F. K. Goodwin, et al. 1988. The NIMH depression awareness, recognition, and treatment program; structure, aims, and scientific basis. *Am. J. Psychiatry,* 145:1351–1357.

Regier, D. A., J. K. Myers, M. Kramer, et al. 1984. The NIMH Epidemiologic Catchment Area program: historical context, major objectives, and study design. *Arch. Gen. Psychiatry,* 41:934–941.

Rice, D., S. Kelman, and L. S. Miller. 1991. Estimates of economic costs of alcohol and drug abuse and mental illness, 1985 and 1988. *Public Health Rep.,* 106:280–292.

Robins, L. N., J. E. Helzer, J. Croughan, et al. 1981. National Institute of Mental Health Diagnostic Interview Schedule: its history, characteristics, and validity. *Arch. Gen. Psychiatry,* 38:381–389.

Robins, L. N., and D. A. Regier, eds. 1991. *Psychiatric Disorders in America—The Epidemiologic Catchment Area Study.* New York: The Free Press.

Shapiro, S., E. A. Skinner, L. G. Kessler, et al. 1984. Utilization of health and mental health services, three Epidemiologic Catchment Area sites. *Arch. Gen. Psychiatry,* 41:971–978.

Shapiro, S., E. A. Skinner, M. Kramer, et al. 1986. Need and demand for mental health services in an urban community: an exploration based on household interviews. In: *Mental Disorders in the Community: Progress and Challenge,* edited by J. Barrett. New York: Guilford Press, pp. 307–320.

Shapiro, S., G. L. Tischler, L. Cottler, et al. 1985. Health services research questions. In: *Epidemiologic Field Methods in Psychiatry: The NIMH Epidemiologic Catchment Area Program,* edited by W. W. Eaton, and L. G. Kessler. Orlando, FL: Academic Press, pp. 191–208.

Shrout, P. E. 1994. The NIMH Epidemiologic Catchment Area program: broken promises and dashed hopes? *Int. J. Methods Psychiatr. Res.,* 4:113–122.

Steinbach, U. 1992. Social networks, institutionalization, and mortality among elderly people in the United States. *J. Gerontol. Soc. Sci.,* 47:S183–S190.

Sudman, S. 1976. *Applied Sampling.* Orlando, FL: Academic Press.

Von Korff, M., L. Cottler, L. K. George, et al. 1985. Nonresponse and nonresponse bias in the ECA surveys. In: *Epidemiologic Field Methods in Psychiatry: The NIMH Epidemiologic Catchment Area Program,* edited by W. W. Eaton, and L. G. Kessler. Orlando, FL: Academic Press, pp. 85–98.

Wolinsky, F., S. D. Culler, C. M. Callahan, et al. 1994. Hospital resource consumption among older adults: a prospective analysis of episodes, length of stay, and charges over a seven-year period. *J. Gerontol. Soc. Sci.,* 49:S240–S252.

Wolinsky, F., and R. J. Johnson. 1991. The use of health services by older adults. *J. Gerontol. Med. Sci.,* 46:S345–S357.

Yaffe, R., S. Shapiro, R. R. Fuchsberg, et al. 1978. Medical economics survey-methods study: cost-effectiveness of alternative survey strategies. *Med. Care,* 16:641–659.

CHAPTER 7

Case Investigation

HAROUTUNE K. ARMENIAN

Major gastrointestinal bleeding following the ingestion of a new analgesic in a 45-year-old woman may be the initial observation that identifies this side effect for the new analgesic.

It is unusual to see an 85-year-old man who has survived the onset of his lung cancer by 23 years since the median survival following diagnosis is less than 1 year. The investigation of this individual may provide clues to the factors affecting long-term survival with lung cancer.

A complaint of mismanagement by a 25-year-old gynecology patient during her hospital stay needs to be reviewed and evaluated by the appropriate hospital authority.

To evaluate the quality of care delivered to patients with hypertension in its outpatient clinics, a health maintenance organization decides to review the records of a sample of patients who have been identified as having hypertension in these clinics.

The professor of surgery in a major teaching hospital would like to review the records of patients treated for gall bladder disease as part of an effort to assess the management issues related to the introduction of laparoscopic cholecystectomy for treating gall bladder disease in that hospital.

These are some examples of problems that require investigation of a case or a series of cases. In many situations in the health services, evaluative judgment is based on data from a case or a series of cases. It is important to understand the process of decision-making under such circumstances and to be familiar with approaches that systematize the information-gathering and inferential processes. This chapter has the following aims:

1. To describe an approach to case investigation in epidemiology and to identify opportunities where it will be a useful way to investigate a problem
2. To assess a report about the investigation of a case and to explain the inferential limitations
3. To explain the strengths and weakness of case investigations in assessing a health problem

Understanding the methods of investigating cases or case series is important because observations from such investigations are often the first step in the process of identifying an important public health or health services problem. These investigations also help develop plausible hypotheses about the etiology of a problem and occasionally provide an explanation for an unusual situation. Understanding the confluence of relevant factors in a single case or series may help us define the problem and its components more accurately.

Theory and Uses of Case Investigation

A case investigation is based on an in-depth study of a single person with a health problem and the facts and events surrounding that person (Armenian, 1991). A case investigation allows the health professional to study the individual as a whole. It is an integrated approach to the multiple determinants of the problem in the individual person, it defines the issues broadly within the context of the particular case, and it gathers information from a variety of sources (Yin, 1993). Thus, a case investigation works by integrating and synthesizing information.

A case investigation in a clinical situation is generally targeted to provide an explanation for the problem being investigated. These are problems that need to be explained in and for themselves, i.e., why and how a patient hospitalized in the coronary care unit developed septicemia due to a common strain of *Staphylococcus* or why a 34-year-old man developed cancer of the rectum. Such questions, dealing with the problems faced by individual patients, need to be answered separately from the broader questions of the routes of transmission of *Staphylococcus* or the epidemiology of colorectal cancer in the general population.

Of necessity, a case investigation is multidisciplinary in approach. In addition to clinical case management, case investigation is extensively used in the social sciences. There is a vast literature in anthropology, psychology, and sociology that is based on case study techniques and the use of both qualitative and quantitative methods of data collection to study such cases. In our discussion in this chapter, we incorporate some of the case study methods used by social scientists in addition to epidemiologic approaches. Table 7-1 lists situations where a case investigation is of value in the health sciences.

Epidemiologists are involved in the investigation of single cases in a number

Table 7-1. Uses of case investigation methods

Etiologic research
Pathology investigation
Clinical case investigation
Medicolegal or product liability cases
Genetics
Occupational medicine
Medical social work
Administration

of situations. These include routine investigation of case reports of common reportable conditions in health departments and assessment of a disease that is rare or unusual in character. Examples of the first type of inquiry include investigation of the contacts of a case of tuberculosis or of a case of sexually transmitted disease. A case of rectal cancer in a 34-year-old man is rare and worthy of investigation since most cases of colorectal cancer occur in persons over the age of 60 years. The latter may be an example of an unusual or rare case.

Although a number of case studies in management and social sciences are done for descriptive purposes, a case investigation, as discussed in this chapter, is used as a tool for etiologic studies, albeit sometimes of an exploratory nature. Although a case investigation may start as a descriptive activity, it has a definite explanatory purpose. We may obtain a descriptive profile of the personal characteristics of the 34-year-old man with the rectal cancer, but the epidemiologic case investigation aims at explaining why he developed the cancer. Thus, the approaches that we need to use may involve techniques that go beyond the regular clinical investigation and its routine data-gathering process.

In general, we are interested, in a case investigation, in the following situations:

1. To study a problem that is of serious concern for a patient or a client of the health services system. In this type of approach, the primary concern of the investigation is to explain the occurrence of the problem in the individual patient. Here, the investigation could be of direct benefit to the patient. For example, it is important to explain why Mr. XP developed an acute myocardial infarction. The presence of coronary heart disease risk factors in this patient may guide us through a management process that may help us develop future preventive strategies for Mr. XP.

2. To investigate an unusual *outlier* (a person whose profile does not fit an established pattern for the condition under investigation). Such an investigation may shed light on the etiologic process for the condition in general. For example, in an outbreak of food-borne illness following a social func-

tion of the Ladies' Guild, Mr. K is the only male in this outbreak involving mostly middle-aged women. Mr. K consumed food that was brought home from this social function by his wife. Through a case investigation it is possible to identify the food item brought home by his wife as the potential culprit causing the outbreak. Being the only male with the disease made Mr. K an outlier. The investigation of his illness may lead us to develop a specific hypothesis as to the food item that was causing the outbreak since he was exposed to only one food item and became sick, while the other patients had the opportunity to be exposed to a number of additional food items.

3. To investigate a typical, or a representative, case of a group of persons with a similar problem. Usually, such a study aims at obtaining preliminary information about the category of persons and at identifying some common characteristics involving a subgroup. Such an investigation is also useful to develop investigative instruments for a larger study of the group as a whole. A case of staphylococcal septicemia may be studied as representative of all similar cases with the condition to identify, for example, the limitations of the information-gathering process with the larger population of cases or for getting some leads to the etiology of staphylococcal septicemia under such circumstances. Within the context of outbreak investigation, the initial attempt at laboratory isolation of the agent may focus on a few selected cases. Similarly, initial laboratory investigations in a prevalent disease of unknown etiology may select a few representative cases to test for a variety of suspected agents.

Thus, case investigations are useful at two levels: at the level of the case, the investigation aims at providing as complete an explanation as possible of the etiology of the specific problem affecting the case, while at the group level, the case investigation can provide important leads to the etiology of the condition in general.

Examples of Specific Uses of the Case Investigation Approach

Clinical case investigation

The investigation of a clinical case may address a number of questions: What is the diagnosis of the patient? What is the best approach for the management of this case? What are the severity of the condition and the prognosis in this patient? Clinical case investigation tries to explain the reason(s) why this particular person developed the disease. The primary reason for the investigation is the welfare of the individual patient. Thus, clinical case investigation also generates data that are essential to an evaluation of the management the patient is receiving. Case investigations also help in the identification of the etiology and the mode of acquisition of disease in the individual patient. For example, it is important to determine whether an unexplained renal failure in a woman is due to exposures from within her workplace. In such circumstances, the epidemiologist-clinician uses prior knowledge about the risk factors and the etiology of the disease to explain the occurrence of the incident event. To explain the case of renal failure based on the clinical information, one develops a number of hypotheses (diagnoses) and tries to gather the evidence for or against these hypotheses. One may, for example, review exposure to various chemicals in the workplace to identify potential toxins. Using actual records, it may be possible to delimit the exposure of the case to these toxins by detailed work histories.

Pathologic investigation

A favorite of generations of physicians, clinicopathologic case reports combine information about the clinical data and a review of the pathology of the same individual. Case studies in pathology

> should do more than document the rare and the unusual. At its best a case study should present observations that tend to test, support, or refute some current principle or hypothesis, resolve a polemic, or explain an unexpected observation. (Kraus, 1991)

Beyond the medicolegal autopsy, the pathologist is able to explain the pathogenesis in a number of clinical situations. Identification of the etiologic agent within samples and tissue obtained from the patient is just one of the roles of the pathologist investigating a case. The spread of the disease in the individual as well as other parameters allow the formulation of a prognosis in addition to an etiologic assessment of the case.

Medicolegal or product liability cases

The primary concern of these cases is to establish beyond reasonable doubt a relation between the development of a disease or other adverse outcome and exposure to a product, process, or caregiver. In such circumstances, it is important to understand the differences in the rules of evidence between criminal law and epidemiology. Evans (1978) has made a comparison between evidence in criminal law and disease causation and has identified many similarities in the principles involved. Within the medicolegal environment of liability cases, we are interested in assessing causation at the individual case level rather than in demonstrating a general etiologic relation between exposure and disease. The relevance of information from the group studies to the individual person is an issue that needs to be addressed in such cases.

Genetics

A large number of associations have been established between genetic factors and a number of diseases using case investigations. For example, statistical analysis of a pedigree in a family allows us to make inferences about the probability of the disease being genetic and the possible mode of inheritance. The availability of well-established protocols in the study of diseases suspected to be genetic has allowed major progress to be made in this field. With the expansion of techniques of DNA analysis, case investigation will take on a new dimension in genetic epidemiology.

Occupational risk assessment

Persons working in industry need to be informed if they have a higher risk for disease because of occupational exposure. Monitoring and surveillance of disease outcomes in individual workers is an important activity for occupational medicine. Risk has to be assessed at the personal level beyond estimates of probability based on data about the group. A worker exposed to asbestos runs a higher risk for mesothelioma if he is also a cigarette smoker. The assessment of his personal risk for the cancer has to take into consideration the fact that he is a smoker, the duration of his exposure, its dose, etc. In another example, it may be important to determine whether hepatic damage in a worker of a chemical factory is due to exposures within the workplace. Based on the clinical information, we develop a number of hypotheses (diagnoses) and gather the evidence for or against them. We also may study the chemical processes involved in the industry to identify the potential hepatotoxins within the workplace that may be related to the liver disease.

Medical social work and health services administration

Social workers and medical administrators are involved in case investigation on a continuous basis. Cases come to the attention of administrators and social workers for a number of problems or complaints. It is important that the professionals dealing with these problems have an understanding of the determinants of the problems in the individual patient.

From the unusual event to the regular clinical patient, the use of case investigation methods helps us in problem-solving for the individual person as well as in understanding some of the determinants of the health problem that is of concern to the group. The next section presents some approaches to case investigation.

Steps in the Process of Case Investigation

The epidemiologic skills for case investigation are different from those needed in a population-based study. Some of these skills are derived from clinical medicine, while others may use in-depth probing techniques developed in the social sciences. The most common approach for learning these skills in epidemiology has been experiential. This chapter provides a conceptual framework to a method that has remained mostly nonstructured in the practice of epidemiology.

A number of approaches to case investigation have been used traditionally by practicing epidemiologists. The study of the initial cases or the rare cases in an outbreak is one situation where approaches can be identified in case investigation. Epidemiologists have used a number of lead questions to investigate the etiology of a case in the absence of established protocols. An example of current guidelines for conducting an interview of reportable cases by epidemiologists was prepared at the Maryland Department of Health and Mental Hygiene. Following is an excerpt:

- Determine a general outline of the information you want to obtain
- Eliminate distractions
- Go to private but safe location for personal interview
- Think of all the possibilities; formulate hypotheses and ask questions that will refute the hypotheses—not just those that support them
- Ask open ended questions if you are "exploring"
- Listen for a "picture"; don't assume things; keep asking until the picture is clear
- Know when to stop the interview (Dwyer, 1991, p. 1)

Well-tested protocols for case investigation in the social sciences, clinical medicine, and genetics allow us to describe a multidisciplinary approach in the investigation of a case.

The process of inquiry into the etiology of a case should not be arbitrary. Organized protocols can enhance the yield and efficiency from such case investigations (Armenian, 1991). There is a wealth of information to collect from a case. Thus, it is possible to introduce a large number of variables in the analysis. Also, we are not limited to a single source of data collection in a case investigation, and such data could be both qualitative and quantitative. It is estimated that, on average, about 500 elements of data are collected for every case studied clinically (Albert et al., 1988). Thus, for a number of clinical case situations, we can start with a rich existing data base.

It is important to define at the outset the objectives of the case investigation. This also will allow the formulation of a few hypotheses to explain the phenomenon under consideration. As in other problem-solving approaches, definition of the study objectives is also a step toward defining, at the outset, the boundaries of the problem under consideration. For example, are we investigating a hypertensive patient to identify a specific risk profile or to get a better understanding of the factors involved in the compliance of such patients to a drug regimen in general? Defining the objectives of the case investigation will help us to define a hypothesis that will be tested by our investigation.

The framework within which most case investigations are conducted is one of problem-solving rather than generating fundamental knowledge. Thus, like any other type of empiric research, case investigation must involve a phase of study design, a process of data collection, data analysis, and reporting of findings (Yin, 1993). As such, a case investigation has to incorporate all of the steps of a research design. The design will force the investigator to define the objectives of the investigation and to develop methods of data collection, analysis, and interpretation. Thus, a case investigation, like other research activities, has to have a well-defined research plan. A research design aims at ensuring that the logical framework is the basis for conducting the investigation and is maintained throughout its implementation.

As listed in Table 7-2, the following are some proposed steps in conducting a case investigation.

Problem delineation

At this first stage of our investigation, we are concerned with delineating clearly the boundaries of the problem our investigation is tackling. Are we concerned primarily with the specific issues of the individual patient or some broader issue regarding a category of patients? Are we aiming at learning something new about the underlying disease or the problem in its general context? As stated previously, our design is going to be different, depending on how we define our problem.

Defining a hypothesis

A hypothesis will provide direction to our investigation. In a case of liver cancer that we are trying to explain based on our antecedent knowledge about the

Table 7-2. Steps in a case investigation

Define the problem and purpose of the investigation
Develop the hypothesis(es) to be tested
Provide an identity to the case
Develop (or decide on) the data collection methods and instruments
Collect the data as planned
Develop a synthesis of the data collected and organize it in a logical framework
Make the appropriate inferences as to the original hypothesis(es)

etiology of the disease, we develop a number of hypotheses. Thus, if our case is an employee in a chemical company, the occupational exposure hypothesis is plausible, but we need to consider other hypotheses such as food exposure to aflatoxins or hepatitis B. In the development of these hypotheses, we start by ruling out artifacts as potential explanatory factors for the problem under consideration. For example, could there be measurement error or diagnostic misclassification in arriving at the diagnosis of liver cancer?

Data collection

Listing the various hypotheses and the priorities established among them will dictate the data needs of our investigation. We may start by collecting data that reject or support the most probable hypothesis, followed by data to test the alternative hypotheses. A sudden, unexpected death in the hospital may be due to the underlying disease of the patient (most probable hypothesis), the personal risk profile and antecedents of the patient (alternative hypothesis 1), factors related to inadequate medical care (alternative hypothesis 2), and possible foul play (alternative hypothesis 3). The investigation of such an unexpected death in the hospital will lead us to gather information about the severity and progress of the underlying disease, the personal characteristics of the patient, the treatments and procedures that the patient underwent in the hospital, and, if suspected, possible sources of foul play. Data collection will start from the most plausible and could move in a stepwise manner to the least plausible hypothesis. Thus, data collection in a case investigation may involve a sequential approach whereby data about one hypothesis are not collected until a more prioritized hypothesis is ruled out. Such an approach may provide some increase in efficiency.

Synthesis

This is a stage in case investigation that organizes information from a variety of sources into a rational framework for decision-making. A simple approach is to match the data to the hypotheses to which they relate. This will help in making separate judgments about each of the hypotheses. The aim of synthesis is not organizational only; we hope to establish through such a process linkages between the various pieces of data. In the process of establishing such linkages, it is likely that we will make observations about associations that have not been hitherto recognized. It is important to consider a case as a whole system. Our approach in case investigation is not atomistic, whereby we are trying to dissect a relation between a subcomponent and a single factor. Our approach is more holistic. The framework of our study, our universe for investigation, is the single case and what goes on around it.

Inferences

These steps in case investigation provide us with a framework that is very general and broad (Table 7-3). It is important to see these steps as a continuum and that every step of the process links with what has been observed previously to find out whether a logical sequence and consistency are maintained.

A case investigation is a dynamic process whereby progress in a particular aspect may guide us to move beyond our initial plans in data collection. There is also a dynamic interaction between progress and the methods used for data collection.

Inferential Approaches

Our approach to making inferences from a case investigation may be different from that used in a study of a group of persons. The case investigation does not

Table 7-3. Elements of systematic data collection in case investigation

Orient the case as to *time, place,* and *personal* characteristics. We may need to start a case investigation by using systematic probing techniques about time, place, and personal characteristics. The season of occurrence, diurnal changes, possible latency, geographic locale and mobility, personal habits, demographic characteristics, and social and occupational histories are some of the data elements of interest.

Use *standardized questionnaires.* These are questionnaires that will collect standard data about the epidemiologic characteristics of the case or some relevant information within the context of testing a particular hypothesis. For example, standard questionnaires about life events may help to identify unusual exposures and events in a case and may help to place or identify etiologic exposures. Such questionnaires will help to establish benchmarks in the life history of the case, around which a variety of potential exposures could be localized and studied.

Conduct relevant *biologic investigations.* These may be dictated by the nature of the pathology under consideration, to establish the appropriate linkages with specific exposures.

Investigate the *family and other small groups* around the case. A detailed family history, sometimes with a genealogic chart and a history of past illnesses and use of medications, is a must for a number of case investigations.

In the rare case situation, study the *unusual experiences* of the individual. The assumption is that an unusual disease occurrence may result from an unusual set of circumstances. Sometimes the nature of the exposure itself may be usual, but the circumstances or dose of exposure may be uncommon.

Inquire into the *likes* and the *dislikes* of the individual to gain insight into the etiology of the case. Identification of hobbies may lead to knowledge of a peculiar behavior that may have led to a harmful exposure or experience.

Source: Armenian (1991).

aim at establishing all possible etiologies for the condition; our primary objective is to explain the outcome in the particular individual. The case is a defined universe, and the inferences we make refer primarily to an explanation pertaining to the individual. We are not necessarily aiming at explaining all phenomena of a similar nature. We may use the information generated from the study of the individual case to explain other similar cases, but our primary objective is to provide as comprehensive an explanation for the problem under consideration in this case as possible (Armenian, 1991).

During the process of making inferences from the data generated about the case, the criteria or postulates for causation may have as much relevance to case investigation as to research in groups of persons. The brief review that follows assesses the usefulness of the Henle-Koch postulates and the standard criteria for judgment as a framework to assess a causal association during a case investigation.

The first postulate of Henle-Koch states that a certain parasite occurs in every case of a disease and that the pathologic changes observed are consistent with the presence of the parasite. In a case investigation, we must demonstrate the presence of the parasite or the exposure in the patient. Demonstration of the appropriate pathology in the presence of the exposure is a requirement at the level of the individual case and represents an advantage of case investigation as a method. In traditional case investigations, epidemiologists have aimed at establishing topographic concordance of pathology and etiology. The occurrence of skin cancer at the site of burns caused by heating with Kangri pots in northern India around the turn of the century led to reports of an association of this type of cancer with the burns.

The second postulate deals with the fact that the parasite should not be present in any other disease in "a fortuitous and nonpathogenic" form. In a case investigation, the presence of another agent that could explain the case is strongly against a causal explanation.

The third postulate is concerned with replicating the disease following exposure to the parasite or the suspected agent. We may satisfy this postulate for a case investigation when we demonstrate that the patient has developed the disease following exposure to a known etiologic agent. In a number of situations where disease is recurrent and episodic, as in an atopic model of etiology, recurrence of the condition may be demonstrated following repeated exposure to the agent (see "Case Reviews," below, for an example).

As with the Henle-Koch postulates, the standard criteria for judgment for a causal association are relevant in establishing an etiologic relation in a case investigation. Thus, time sequence is a most powerful criterion for such investigations. If we are unable to demonstrate antecedence of exposure to the onset of the disease, then our efforts at satisfying all other criteria are no longer useful. In case investigations, we look for sequential linkage of suspected exposure to the onset of the disease process, especially when the occurrence of the disease is associated with a new and unusual event in the patient's life.

Strength of the association is another criterion that needs to be adapted. Strength could be satisfied if the pathology produced as a result of exposure to the suspected agent is very serious and debilitating. Similarly, dose response in a case could be a reflection of the severity of the pathology as the dose of exposure increases. Considering that for the individual case there may be fewer suspected exposures than for a group of cases, specificity as a criterion may be easier to satisfy. The biologic plausibility of the association has to be established with the same rigor in the case investigation as in a group. The investigator needs to inquire whether the suspected etiology in this case provides a coherent and (as much as possible) complete explanation of the occurrence of the disease.

In making inferences, the investigator regards replication as the most relevant criterion for causation. Replication is the logical framework upon which our judgment is based in making inferences, as was discussed above for a particular subset of recurrent illnesses. However, we may be interested also in demonstrating a replication of findings from a number of case investigations.

Standard population-based group studies use sampling logic. Sampling logic assumes "that an investigation is mainly interested in 'representing' a larger universe" (Yin, 1993, p. 39). Case studies follow a replication approach. As stated by Yin (1993, p, 34):

> two or more cases should be included within the same study precisely because the investigator predicts that similar results (replications) will be found. If such replications are indeed found for several cases, you can have more confidence in the overall results. The development of consistent findings, over multiple cases and even multiple studies, can then be considered a very robust finding.

Traditionally, epidemiologists using case investigations have tried first to identify, in the specific case, exposure to agents that are established etiologic factors in other diseases with a similar pathology.

Epidemiology is interested in the investigation of cases that both support and refute the hypothesis. When a large majority of cases support the hypothesis and very few outliers do not, we may need to identify alternative explanations to the prevailing one to untangle the etiologic relation.

One of the approaches in case investigation is sequential data gathering. Sufficient data are collected to allow reasonable conclusions about a hypothesis that best fits all of the information. Thus, it is important for the investigator to decide at the outset the level of uncertainty he or she is willing to accept in making a decision about the relation being investigated. As stated previously, the most efficient approach is the one that tests sequentially a series of hypotheses of varying levels of plausibility.

The introduction of sociometric methods in epidemiology over the past six decades has deemphasized case-based investigations. The concern for predicting the occurrence of the next case has evolved to approaches that aim at generalizing to, or estimating, an average.

> A fatal flaw in doing case studies is to conceive of statistical generalization as the method of generalizing the results of the case. This is because cases are not "sampling units" and should not be chosen for this reason. . . . Multiple cases, in this sense, should be considered like multiple experiments. . . . Under these circumstances, the method of generalization is "analytic generalization," in which a previously developed theory is used as a template with which to compare the empirical results of the case study. If two or more cases are shown to support the same theory, replication is claimed. The empirical results may be considered more potent if two or more cases support the same theory but do not support an equally plausible rival theory. (Yin, 1993, p. 50)

> The most common rival theory has been the null hypothesis. For doing case study research, the best rival is not simply the absence of the target theory or hypothesis. Instead the best rival would be a rival theory, attempting to explain the same outcome but with a different substantive theory than that of the target theory. If you have rival theories in this sense, you can collect data to test both theories and compare the results through a pattern-matching process. (Yin, 1993, p. 60)

The clinical case investigation essentially uses such an approach of ruling out potential diagnoses by collecting data that would support specific diagnoses or hypotheses. Thus, in a case investigation, we try to systematically refute or challenge current hypotheses by data that could potentially support alternative hypotheses. The investigator tries to falsify the current best explanation on an ongoing basis. This is the approach of making causal inferences that is akin to what was advanced by the philosopher Sir Karl Popper and that is known by his name.

Following is a list of alternative hypotheses that we may consider systematically in a case investigation:

1. There is ascertainment or measurement error. Either the diagnosis or the assessment of the characteristic of interest is wrong.
2. The evidence is in favor of the case being caused by an established risk factor or by a combination of known risk factors.
3. The case is suspected to be caused by a factor that still needs to be established.
4. In the absence of a plausible interpretation, an unusual and rare event could be ascribed to chance.

The next section illustrates by case reviews some of the concepts and approaches that have been discussed so far. Clinical cases are presented first to give examples of approaches that are commonly used in clinical problem-solving and that may be useful for other applications of the method.

Case Reviews

A clinical case

A previously healthy 47-year-old man presented to the emergency room after the sudden onset of cough, shortness of breath, and tightness in his chest while climbing stairs.

George Thibault (1994), the author of this clinical problem-solving report in the *New England Journal of Medicine,* uses this case to illustrate the process of decision-making in a clinical environment as to the appropriateness of level of diagnostic certainty. The problem is summarized in the sentence quoted above. The objective of this case study is that of clinical problem-solving, and as a first step in the process, a reasonable diagnosis for appropriate action must be formulated.

In reviewing the problem statement, an expert clinician lists a diagnosis of acute myocardial ischemia as the first choice (hypothesis) and presents reasons for proposing this diagnosis. ''The chest tightness is especially suggestive of an ischemic episode.'' The clinician makes a qualitative judgment about the nature of the symptoms and identifies it with a pattern that is common to ischemia rather than myocardial infarction. In addition, the clinician lists two other probable diagnoses (cardiac arrhythmia and pulmonary embolism), gives the reasons for these choices, and ends the list with three ''less likely possibilities'': acute myocarditis, acute pericarditis, and acute dissection. Thus, these initial hypotheses or diagnoses are developed on the basis of minimal data, as presented in the first sentence. To arrive at these hypotheses, the expert uses previous knowledge (experience) that is structured and organized in his or her mind in a way that will elicit these options based on a quick judgment applicable to the data at hand.

Based on standard clinical practice, data collection has a well-defined structure and follows a system that starts by getting information from historical antecedents, the events leading to the clinical presentation, the physical examination, and appropriate laboratory tests. With each additional piece of data, the clinician reconsiders the initial hypothesis(es) and evaluates the condition of the patient, to provide the most appropriate management dictated by the information available at that moment. Thus, there is a dynamic interactive system that could be modeled like a spiral. It starts with the problem statement, followed by the development of the hypothesis(es) that leads to the data collection process and that results in two types of result: a reconsideration of the initial hypothesis and the need for therapeutic interventions based on the information available at that point in time. The revised diagnosis and the results of the interventions will lead to a new set of data collection activities, as well as new interventions and a reconsideration of the diagnosis or hypothesis.

However, at each of the stages of data collection there is an effort at synthesis of information and reconsideration of options. Thus, the process of inferences is not a terminal event but is continuously integrated within a continuum, as described above.

In this particular clinical case investigation, the initial history reveals that in the past month the patient had two similar episodes during activity and in "each instance his symptoms resolved slowly over several hours without any intervention other than rest." We also learn that the patient was a smoker of about 20 years but had stopped for the past 5 years and that his "father had died of a myocardial infarction at the age of 63." A review of this information makes the clinician refine the initial primary diagnosis by stating that these "findings are in contrast to the consequences of a long-standing fixed coronary-artery obstruction" and adding to the list of possibilities the unusual diagnosis of left atrial myxoma. From the physical examination in the emergency room, the clinician picks wheezing as the most important finding and considers it compatible with an acute ischemic episode with "transient pulmonary congestion." For the clinician, the most important additional data at this point would be an electrocardiogram. The latter is essentially normal except for "minor nonspecific ST-segment and T-wave changes." Such an observation leads the expert to conclude that it is "less likely that the patient is having a major ischemic episode." However, "the low value for the partial pressure of arterial oxygen makes me think it is more likely that he has had a pulmonary embolus."

In the meantime, the patient is treated in the emergency room "with inhaled bronchodilator and all his symptoms improved." As a result of this response and the previous findings, the patient is treated for asthma and bronchitis. However, the expert/clinician challenges the diagnosis of asthma on the basis of the known fact that "it is unusual for asthma to occur for the first time at 47 years of age" and because of the severity of the respiratory distress. One month after receiving treatment and during the follow-up visit, the pulmonary consultant is not satisfied with the diagnosis of asthma and asks for a ventilation-perfusion scan, an exercise electrocardiogram, and additional pulmonary function tests. As in the emergency room, the patient response to therapy dictates a reconsideration of the diagnosis. An abnormal exercise electrocardiogram makes a cardiac catheterization the next diagnostic examination and is the basis for a change in the therapeutic regimen of the patient by introducing a beta blocker. The consultant-expert disagrees with the recommendation of a cardiac catheterization due to the lack of some specific indications for the procedure. The catheterization is done 2 months later and reveals "normal hemodynamic values and normal coronary arteries. The patient was discharged and advised to continue to use inhaled bronchodilator. The final diagnosis was bronchial asthma."

In his final discussion of this case, the author addresses the original query: What is the appropriate degree of diagnostic certainty?

> Who was right here? The physician who made a tentative diagnosis of asthma and treated the patient for it? The experts who tested until a diagnosis of coronary disease was excluded? This is one of the difficult questions in modern medicine. . . . Two experts considered the risks of uncertainty to be greater than the risks of a high level of certainty, and they ordered more and more tests until uncertainty nearly vanished. Much of the expense of health care is driven by just this kind of reasoning, and even in retrospect it is difficult to know just who was right.

For our purposes, the important messages to learn from this clinical case investigation include the following:

1. The problem setup in a clinical case investigation is complex and varied. Every patient is a unique entity, but our problem-solving process depends on our cumulated clinical experience, which in itself varies from one practitioner to the next.
2. Despite the complexity of the problem context, clinical case investigation uses standard processes of data collection. The purpose of such standardization is to establish benchmarks for comparison of results.
3. The investigation is closely intertwined with decisions about therapeutics and interventions. The whole process is dynamic, whereby hypotheses are established and continuously challenged on the basis of the additional data that are gathered.
4. The response to therapy influences decisions about diagnosis and directs the clinician toward new interventions.

Clinical etiology

> *A 54 year old white female with perennial and seasonal allergic rhinitis presented to the emergency room with nausea, lightheadedness, and throat constriction. Upon examination she was noted to have angioedema of her eyelids, lips, and tongue. She was treated with epinephrine, diphenhydramine, and methylprednisolone.* (Saryan et al., 1995, p. 3)

This patient presents with severe allergic reaction and needs to be managed immediately because of the serious nature of the illness. Identifying the etiology could wait until life-saving measures are taken. The nature of the illness allows us to focus on etiologic factors that are precipitants of such a severe reaction. The following history is obtained:

The patient had a history of allergic reactions to tree nuts first noted when she took a small bite of a pine nut and had some swelling of her tongue and buccal mucosa. The current episode of severe allergic reaction developed within minutes of eating a hors d'oeuvre at a company Christmas party. A coworker inquired from the restaurant and found out that the hors d'oeuvre contained pine nuts. (Saryan et al., 1995, p. 3)

With the antecedent history and the confirmation that the patient ate pine nuts prior to the current episode of severe reaction, it is not difficult to establish an etiologic relation between the pine nuts and the allergic reaction. From the criteria of judgment for a causal association, we can establish antecedence of exposure to the development of the illness, and strength and dose response are obtained by history, the larger amount of the pine nut in the latter episode causing a more severe illness. Probably the strongest argument in favor of this etiologic relation is replication of the occurrence of the same disease episode following exposure to the pine nuts. However, we also need to address the criteria of specificity and biologic plausibility. In this particular case, the authors resort to laboratory tests to address these criteria.

Prick/puncture immediate hypersensitivity skin testing was performed. Positive wheal and flare reactions were obtained to commercial extracts of walnut, almond, pistachio, and hazelnut, but negative to peanut, cashew, Brazil nut and pecan. Since no commercial extract of pine nut was available, an extract was prepared with pine nuts purchased from a local food store. The patient was prick tested on the forearm using a small drop of the pine nut extract together with histamine and saline controls. A positive reaction was obtained consisting of a 6 mm wheal and 50 mm flare. (Saryan et al., 1995, p. 3)

Considering that the skin tests for the other nuts do not provide a level of specificity, the author develops a specific extract and confirms the clinical suspicion by a controlled test. This case is typical of many clinical investigations involving a workup for atopic reactions. It is important to note that it is possible to base the inferential judgment process on the established epidemiologic criteria for causation.

The next case review is selected from the epidemiologic literature and involves an investigation of the first few cases of a major epidemic. Our interest here is to learn from the process of establishing an association from a study of these early cases.

Etiology/outbreak

In October 1989 three patients in New Mexico presented to their doctors with myalgia and eosinophilia. (Hertzman et al., 1990, p. 869)

The following is a presentation of excerpts from the case report on one of these cases.

A previously healthy 44-year-old woman reported transient shortness of breath and cough, followed by increasingly severe muscular aches and weakness. . . . When first examined on September 29, 1989, four weeks after her symptoms began, she appeared to be moderately ill and was afebrile. (Hertzman et al., 1990, p. 869)

She had tender muscles in her abdomen, shoulders, arms, and legs, with mild weakness. Laboratory tests revealed 42% eosinophils in the leukocytes. All laboratory tests to demonstrate a possible etiologic factor for the eosinophilia, like checking for parasitoses, failed to identify such an agent.

Based on observations on two other patients, a history of ingestion of tryptophan was elicited in this patient, starting about 8 weeks prior to the inception of the symptoms. These were the first cases of an epidemic of what was later termed ʻʻeosinophilia myalgia syndrome.ʼʼ Several thousand cases were detected nationwide, and following serial case-control studies, the disease was linked to the ingestion of tryptophan produced by one particular manufacturer following changes that were introduced in the process of product purification.

The lessons to be learned from a study of these cases are the following:

1. It was not necessary to conduct a large-scale study to establish the relation between the ingestion of tryptophan and the disease. In fact, the disease was defined by the exposure to the agent following these first few cases.
2. The association was established because of the chronologic and geographic confluence of these three cases and replication of findings.
3. The fact that the clinical syndrome of eosinophilia and myalgia is relatively rare stimulated the clinicians to be more assertive in their inquiry about possible exposures.
4. None of the potential agents of eosinophilia searched for in the investigation yielded any additional clues to etiology.

Case Study Evaluation

A case study can be an essential component of evaluation in health services. The case in such a situation is a single project or program or a person who is one of a very small number receiving a new therapy or intervention. Thus, situations where a case study is useful in evaluation include the following:

1. As a descriptive tool. One may need to describe the operation of a program or an intervention to assess whether the process is consistent with original plans.

2. As a method to explore the characteristics of a program or project that needs to be evaluated and about which no systematic antecedent information exists.

3. To assess the effect of single-subject trials where, due to a very limited number of cases of a particular disease or during the early phases of a new drug development program, we may embark on such limited trials.

4. As a demonstration project. Prior to the expansion of an intervention to a large number of sites or organizations, we may decide to test the intervention at a single demonstration site. Demonstration projects can be used in the development of health services in a number of situations, such as the introduction of new technologic advances or changes in the existing system.

Every project in health services involves complex interactions of persons, elements, environmental constraints, and resources. Thus, it is difficult to standardize the evaluation of many such projects based on criteria set externally. Every health services project is an intervention with the possibility of producing a different set of outcomes. Thus, evaluations of individual projects are conceptually similar to evaluations of individual patients. A project has to be evaluated as a whole, and, as in the evaluation of the single patient, data from a number of different sources and using a variety of methods need to be used to make the appropriate judgment.

A project can be considered as a single system with its own structure, processes, and outcome(s). We may use such a systems framework to collect data and apply judgment about the project.

> *The Fund for International Development (FID) is interested in having an evaluation of a rehabilitation and physical therapy unit in the country of Bomanda, which it has been partially funding for about 3 years through a private voluntary organization.*

Such an evaluation could take an approach based on ascertaining the outcomes of the care provided by this unit. In such an approach, we would need to develop a population frame, find some study design that collects data from recipients and nonrecipients of the services, and compare the outcomes in the first group with those in the second. Although improved outcomes as a result of the services are the ultimate objective of the FID project, it may take several years before outcomes of such projects could be ascertained. Thus, a shorter-term evaluation of such a project may focus on an assessment of the structure of the rehabilitation and physical therapy unit by ascertaining the personnel, the facilities, and the equipment used. Such a short-term evaluation also could focus on the process of care at the unit by finding out whether the interventions and the methods used are comparable with some well-established standard. Thus, much of the short-term evaluation of such a project may focus on descriptive observations and data.

As in the individual patient, it is very important to provide a synthesis of information from a variety of sources. Such a synthesis would form the basis of judgment about the program or project.

In the final report of the evaluation of the project in Bomanda, the FID would like to receive judgment as to whether the deployment of personnel and use of facilities are according to initial plans and disbursements and whether the techniques used in the program are of an established standard.

Many of the approaches used in case investigation are useful for descriptive project evaluation. We need to delineate the problem, collect data on the basis of a well-defined framework, synthesize the information, and provide the appropriate inferences.

Case Series in Epidemiology and Health Services

Definitions and uses

Health care professionals have routinely used information about series of cases in judgments about factors associated in the etiology and pathogenesis of disease. Case series also have been used for making decisions about the appropriateness of the delivery of medical care. Some of the most commonly used approaches for evaluation of the quality of medical care in the past have been audits of a group of patients which compared the care given to these patients with some standards set by professional bodies.

The case series is a study of a number of persons, typically receiving health care from the same source and having the same outcome or problem. The study is usually based on data collected routinely and systematically by the health care system. As a method, it tries to organize knowledge, identify common characteristics of a group of patients, and provide insights to some specific questions about the pathogenesis of the outcome.

Clinical researchers have used case series to understand the pathogenesis and natural history of a large number of conditions. A study of a series of 588 cases of Kaposi's sarcoma with AIDS will provide valuable descriptive information about this subgroup of the disease and will allow better understanding of the pathogenesis and prognostic factors in these patients. Further, a review of these cases also may provide us with data regarding problems of access to, and appropriateness of, health services for these patients. However, inferences from such case series are very much dependent on an external standard or comparison.

The following are some situations where the case series has been used as a method of study:

1. In quality assurance programs, where on a periodic basis a series of cases of a particular diagnosis or procedure are reviewed, data are abstracted, and the management of these cases is compared with some standards set by professional organizations. A review of the records of all patients admitted with the diagnosis of cholecystitis in hospital X to assess various components of care is an example of such a series.

2. As part of clinical research that is descriptive in nature. The objective for such studies is to describe the characteristics of a particular disease in a more systematic manner than has hitherto been done. The range of such studies extends from descriptive studies of new diseases and syndromes to clinical descriptions of some new observations of well-established disease entities. An example of such a series would be a description of 43 cases of familial Mediterranean fever (FMF) from Kuwait, where no such cases have been previously reported.

3. In ethnographic research of various disease entities and behaviors. In this approach, a study of a number of cases would provide the researcher a "representative" group to understand some common characteristics of persons with the same disease or health problem. Using interviews of a number of case patients with abdominal pain or cough, we may be able to understand the cultural interpretation of the pathogenesis of these conditions or collate descriptive information about the management of such persons in the community where the study is being conducted.

4. Similar to the single case investigation, one of the earliest steps in the investigation of outbreaks involves a study of a series of cases. The traditional approach in outbreak investigation is to start with the index case, identify additional cases, and confirm the presence of an outbreak. The initial case series allows us to embark on an evaluation of the common characteristics of the cases, develop some preliminary hypotheses as to the etiology, identify the at-risk population, and calculate some attack rates.

The advantages of a case series are limited primarily to clinical case material and data already collected for patient care purposes. A number of case series have used within-group comparisons to make inferences. Examples of such case series are described in the first two case reviews, below.

Limitations of case series

The major limitation of the case series is the lack of appropriate controls or comparison groups. This limits the possibility of establishing an etiologic relation. If it is reported that 35% of the 43 cases of FMF in Kuwait were regular users of aspirin, it will be difficult to make any inferences about this observation without knowledge about the frequency of aspirin use in persons without FMF in Kuwait.

Another limitation involves the biases of selection inherent in every case series. The case series usually represents the specific population within which the study has been done. Generalizability of inferences from most case series is very limited. If all 43 reported cases of FMF are identified from hospital discharge reports, then we may expect that many of the mild cases of the disease may be missed in this case series.

Standard epidemiologic methods are based on the comparative method. In a case series, comparisons are made internally or based on external standards. Sometimes the investigator may compare results with the experience from a previously reported case series. An example of a case series where internal comparisons have been productive is a report of 261 cases of acute myocardial infarction admitted to a coronary care unit, where Sawaya et al. (1980) compared a subgroup of 38 cases of myocardial infarction who developed pericarditis with patients from the same series without pericarditis. They reviewed the data to identify factors that were predictive of the occurrence of pericarditis in the early hours of the development of the acute myocardial infarction.

Following are some examples of investigations using the clinical case series.

Case reviews

Epstein-Barr virus in gastric carcinoma (Tokunaga et al., 1993). In this study, the authors aim at determining the frequency of Epstein-Barr virus (EBV) gastric carcinoma in Japanese patients and clarifying the clinicopathologic characteristics of such tumors.

> *EBV-encoded RNA 1* in situ *hybridization was applied to paraffin sections, including the tumor and adjacent gastric tissue, from 999 gastric carcinomas observed in 970 consecutive cases from a large Japanese hospital. EBV involvement occurred in 6.9% of lesions, a significantly lower proportion than was observed in a North American series. Involvement was significantly more frequent among males, in tumors in the upper part of the stomach, and in adenocarcinomas of the moderately differentiated tubular and poorly differentiated solid or medullary types. Almost all carcinomas with marked lymphoid stroma were EBV-positive.*

This report illustrates the uses and limitations of a series of cases.

1. It deals with a very large number of cases of stomach cancer that are available to the investigators through both records and pathology specimens.

2. The study is able to conduct very thorough laboratory assessment of the readily available specimens.

3. Review of the records provides us with a profile of the patient population under investigation.

4. The major problem with this study is the lack of a comparison group of patients with no stomach cancer. The authors compare their results with what was observed in a similar series from North America, but their comparison group is still another series of cases rather than controls. The study of normal tissue from individual cancer patients does not replace the need for nonpathologic controls.

5. The most informative component of the study is when the authors embark on an analysis of their results through internal comparisons. We learn more specifically about the topographic distribution of the EBV-positive lesions and the type of pathology that is more associated with EBV, and we are told that ''almost all carcinomas with marked lymphoid stroma were EBV positive.'' The latter finding is consistent with our previous knowledge of the association of EBV with lymphoid malignancies and diseases involving the lymphatic system, such as infectious mononucleosis.

6. Our ability to generalize from the results of this study is limited because of the selection of cases from a single hospital. Do these results apply to stomach cancer cases in Japan in general? We need additional data to answer this question. The large size of the sample (case series) does not protect the study from selection bias.

In summary, this investigation of a series of cases is useful as a descriptive study only, and our ability to make inferences from the data presented is limited to within-group comparisons.

Studies of amyotrophic lateral sclerosis in Sardinia, southern Italy (Rosati et al., 1977). Amyotrophic lateral sclerosis (ALS), a neurologic motor neuron disease, has been studied extensively by clinicians and epidemiologists in an attempt to understand its etiology. In this particular study, from the island of Sardinia, the authors identified all 125 cases that were initially diagnosed as ALS over a 10-year period. These cases were identified from all available sources of information, including hospital and insurance records and outpatient facilities. Following a review of the records, 96 were finally accepted as ALS patients and, in 29, the initial diagnosis was rejected.

Based on the available information and denominator data about the population of Sardinia, the authors were able to calculate annual incidence rates for ALS, as well as incidence rates for different age, sex, and occupational categories. However, for the different characteristics that had no denominator information, they calculated relative frequencies. Following is an excerpt from the abstract of this paper:

ALS started on average at 56.58 years and its duration was 2.5 years, being significantly longer in patients under 40-year-old. The distribution of the various clinical forms was: 66 per cent conventional forms, 20 per cent bulbar, and 14 per cent pseudo-polyneuritic. In the bulbar type, a female predominance was found. About 96 per cent of cases were sporadic and 4 per cent familial. Familial cases presented no difference from sporadic cases. Trauma was present in 10.5 per cent of the cases and gastrointestinal disfunction in 13 per cent. This probably reflects some relationship between trauma and ALS, and between malnutrition and ALS. No combination of ALS, dementia and parkinsonism was observed. Dementia was associated with ALS in four cases and Parkinson's disease in one case, separately. The combination of other disease states with ALS in the present study may be simple coincidence. (Rosati et al., 1977)

A review of this report of a series of cases of ALS helps us make the following observations:

1. The major strength of this case series compared with other series is that the study is population-based. The investigators have a well-defined population of reference that allows them to calculate incidence rates on the basis of census information about demographic characteristics. However, when such information is not available at the population level, the authors are limited in their inferences.
2. As in the previous case series, this study is able to make some internal comparisons, such that familial cases were no different from sporadic cases or the finding of female predominance in the bulbar subtype of the disease.
3. The authors have carefully reviewed the data about each of the cases and validated the diagnoses. Measurement of outcome and data could be as rigorous in case series as in other research methods.
4. The major limitation of this case series is the same for all similar studies: the absence of a comparison group. There are a number of instances in this study where the authors try to make etiologic inferences with some of their observations, but they are limited because of the absence of a comparison group. The significance of the observations of a history of trauma in 10.5% of these patients and gastrointestinal dysfunction in 13% cannot be interpreted with the available information. However, additional case information—for example, about the nature of the trauma on a case-by-case basis—may have improved the information value of this observation. In another series of 35 cases of ALS from the Mayo Clinic, the authors describe three patients who developed ALS following trauma. The weakness of the ALS started in the same extremity as the trauma within 3 months to 3 years following the injury. Such additional data about the

cases, establishing topographic concordance between the suspected etiologic factor and the site of the pathology, make a trauma hypothesis more
plausible.

This paper further highlights the importance of a comparison group of controls in establishing etiologic associations. Because of such limitations of the case
series, the method of choice for studying associations under such circumstances
is case-control. With some additional effort, the authors of this report could have
developed a control group of non-ALS persons, and their ability to make inferences from this study may have improved dramatically.

Evaluating the appropriateness of care: a study of cesarean section rates
(Kazandjian and Summer, 1989). Our third example presents data from the
quality assurance literature.

The dramatic rise in rates of cesarean sections (C-section) over the past two
decades has raised questions about the appropriateness of a large number of these
operations. Reliance on this surgical mode of delivery has escalated from 4.5% in
1965 to 24.1% in 1986 and is expected to be 40.3% by the year 2000 if the current
trends continue. A "number of reasons have been suggested for the increased
C-section rates, including physician training, complications of labor, patient
preferences, and physicians' fear of litigation" (Kazandjian and Summer, 1989).

In addressing this issue of high C-section rates in the state, the Council for
Quality of Health Care of the Maryland Hospital Association, having reviewed
the available official data on hospital-specific C-section rates, "concluded that
existing data on hospitals' overall C-section rates and rates of primary and repeat
C-sections were useful only for initial screening purposes." The council established an obstetrics advisory committee (OAC) "to gather the necessary data to
investigate the C-section rate and to design, test, practically apply, and validate a
set of guidelines (protocol) that would assist hospitals in internal peer review of
C-sections." Following an extensive review process of existing guidelines and
protocols, "it became readily apparent that a C-section review protocol that could
be used by all hospitals was needed as a first step in developing a tool for
monitoring and evaluating the appropriateness of C-sections." The protocol of
data collection that was developed was pilot tested at six hospitals. There were
important differences among the hospitals as to the presence of recorded data
about all elements needed by the protocol. The protocol was modified accordingly (Kazandjian and Summer, 1989).

The results section of this study presents a tabulation of the percentage of
records with selected characteristics, based on the protocol set by the OAC,
which focused on the process of care, such as whether there was an attempt at
vaginal delivery (2–12% of the records in the various hospitals), and on patient

and fetal response, such as whether there were any signs of fetal distress (10–38%) or complications of pregnancy (10–25%). The authors also present coefficients of variation for selected C-section characteristics among these six hospitals. The highest interhospital variation was for the attempt at vaginal delivery, and the lowest was for the presence of a fetal monitor. In the last section of this paper, the authors discuss the potential for generalizing the process, particularly that of developing a consensus.

This paper presents a description of the process of developing a review protocol for a problem in the assessment of quality of care. The steps that were discussed involved an appreciation of the importance of the problem to be evaluated; the development of accepted guidelines on standards of care, whether these are based on the process or the structure of the system; data collection and analysis; inferences; and recommended intervention. Following are some differences between the review of a series of cases in a quality assurance (QA) program like this and the clinical case series discussed previously.

1. The review of records in QA is based on some established external standard of care. These external standards are based on either consensus within a professional group (in the current study) or research that supports the necessity of setting such a standard. Thus, although there may be no control group in such a review, the care of the patient is compared with some external standard. Such an approach makes the inferential process easier than in the absence of a comparison group.
2. Because the data collection process in most QA programs uses some previously established standard protocols, it is possible to conduct comparisons with data about the same health problem from other hospitals. Thus, comparisons in a case series in a QA program are not as much of a problem as in clinical case series.

Conclusions

We have discussed two approaches of investigation frequently used in the delivery of health services. The case investigation and the case series have well-defined uses in epidemiologic investigation, provided we are aware of their limitations.

Both of these approaches are useful for making an initial description of the characteristics of the problem context and for developing initial hypotheses about the factors responsible for the problem. However, if concern is limited to the universe of the individual case or case series under investigation, then some of the approaches discussed here may facilitate the making of appropriate inferences.

The conduct of a case investigation or a study of a series of cases should not compromise the scientific rigor of the data collection process and the systematic approach to analysis and to the inferential process. Some of the same principles and methods that apply to population-based epidemiologic investigations are relevant to case investigation or case series.

References

Albert, D. A., R. Munson, and M. D. Resnik. 1988. *Reasoning in Medicine*. Baltimore: Johns Hopkins University Press.

Armenian, H. K. 1991. Case investigation in epidemiology. *Am. J. Epidemiol.*, 134: 1067–1072.

Dwyer, D. M. 1991. *Communicating and Interviewing*. Baltimore: Epidemiology and Disease Control Program, Maryland Department of Health and Mental Hygiene.

Evans, A. S. 1978. Causation and disease: a chronological journey. *Am. J. Epidemiol.*, 108:249–258.

Hertzman, P. A., W. L. Blevins, J. Mayer, et al. 1990. Association of the eosinophilia-myalgia syndrome with the ingestion of tryptophan. *N. Engl. J. Med.*, 322:869–873.

Kazandjian, V. A., and S. J. Summer. 1989. Evaluating the appropriateness of care: a study of cesarean section rates. *Qual. Rev. Bull.*, 15:206–214.

Kraus, F. T. 1991. Case studies, case reports, and human pathology. *Hum. Pathol.*, 22:735–736.

Rosati, G., L. Pinna, E. Granieri, et al. 1977. Studies on epidemiological, clinical, and etiological aspects of ALS disease in Sardinia, southern Italy. *Acta Neurol. Scand.*, 55:231–244.

Saryan, J. A., A. Bouras, and J. M. O'Loughlin. 1995. Anaphylaxis to pine nuts hidden in restaurant food [Abstract]. In: *Proceedings of the Sixth Armenian Medical World Congress*. July 5–9, 1995, Boston, MA.

Sawaya, J. I., S. K. Mujais, and H. K. Armenian. 1980. Early diagnosis of pericarditis in acute myocardial infarction. *Am. Heart J.*, 100:144–151.

Thibault, G. E. 1994. The appropriate degree of diagnostic certainty. *N. Engl. J. Med.*, 331:1216–1220.

Tokunaga, M., C. E. Land, Y. Uemura, et al. 1993. Epstein-Barr virus in gastric carcinoma. *Am. J. Pathol.*, 143:1250–1254.

Yin, R. K. 1993. *Applications of Case Study Research*. Newbury Park, CA: Sage Publications.

CHAPTER 8

Case-Control Methods

HAROUTUNE K. ARMENIAN

A Problem-Solving Tool

The high cost and complex logistics of conducting randomized experimental studies make them difficult to develop routinely to evaluate the delivery of health care. In addition to cost and logistics, there are other problems in setting up a randomized trial. For example, it is difficult to assess a problem as complex as an alternative system of delivery of medical care using a randomized trial, and it is difficult to justify a randomized clinical trial if efficacy is already established and our primary concern in evaluating an intervention is its adverse effects. In both instances, well-designed observational studies may provide an alternative to randomized clinical trials. Table 8-1 lists some of the situations where an alternative approach to randomized trials should be considered.

Of the observational epidemiologic study designs, the case-control method is the most efficient to use in the evaluation of health services. It allows us to get a relatively quick answer to the question under consideration at minimal cost. By contrast, clinical trials are long and expensive. Take, for example, the high cost of medical care as a problem requiring study. The Rand Study (Newhouse, 1974; Brook et al., 1983) was an experiment where people were assigned at random to different systems of health care and the effects of these systems on health outcomes as well as costs were studied (see Chapter 9). Since the completion of that study in 1982, no other randomized study has been conducted to test similar hypotheses.

The key attribute of a case-control design is the comparison of two groups: one with a specific outcome and the other without that outcome. The frequency of the hypothesized factor(s) suspected to be related to the outcome is compared in these two groups. If the outcome of interest is an adverse effect of a particular treatment, then the cases will be persons with the adverse effect and the controls will be those who do not have the adverse effect. The two groups will be compared as to the frequency of exposure to the suspected treatment. Because of its

Table 8-1. Situations where alternatives to randomized trials may need to be considered

---

The outcome being studied is very rare.

The ethical climate is not conducive for a second randomized trial. There are ethical constraints for conducting randomized trials, such as potential major side effects of the intervention or evidence that one of the alternative interventions has advantages.

The disease to be prevented or the outcome to be affected has a latency period spanning several years and decades.

The intervention under review is available and of widespread use in the community.

We need to study potential side effects of a particular intervention.

Following the establishment of efficacy, we have to assess the impact of an intervention within the community.

---

focus on explaining the occurrence of various outcomes, the case-control method is well suited to health services research (Selby, 1994).

Although the gold standard for evaluating an alternative approach to the delivery of medical care is the randomized trial, the case-control method may provide information for a host of decisions within the framework of health services. Whether these decisions involve issues of etiology, efficacy, effectiveness, or efficiency, the case-control method can be useful (Armenian and Lilienfeld, 1994; Comstock, 1994; Greenland et al., 1981; Selby, 1994).

Also, the case-control method may be useful at each of the steps in the problem-solving process, from defining the problem to assessing its key determinants, to quantifying risk or evaluating intervention strategies, and to setting policy priorities. As an investigative tool, it is one of the most frequently used methods in health studies. For many problems, it allows the efficient ascertainment of associations between an outcome and determinants of that outcome.

Defining the outcome

A problem is an outcome that we would like to avoid or prevent, such as increased death rates from lung cancer, disability from osteoarthritis, or measles in a community where vaccines are available. Metastatic breast cancer where mammographic services are obtainable or very high-cost medical care in a subset of patients within a population are other problems that could be studied using the case-control method. This method compels us first to define explicitly the outcome or the problem. Such a definition would facilitate greatly one of the earlier steps of the method, that of defining the cases. If our interest is to investigate the problem of measles in a population that has access to vaccination, then cases must be selected from the same population and ages or from subgroups that are targeted by the current practice of vaccination. Thus, in a particular population where measles vaccines have been available over the past three decades, cases will include all medically diagnosed measles cases in persons less than 25 years old. If we want to undertake an investigation of the problem of disability in osteo-arthritis, then we need to specify our understanding of disability to arrive at a definition of the cases. For example, cases may be defined as patients with osteoarthritis who are unable to perform independently daily chores of personal care. Thus, the definition of a case in a case-control study forces us to delineate better and to be more specific about the problem we are investigating.

Identifying a comparison group

To learn about the key determinants of the problem under consideration, we use the case-control method to compare cases who have the outcome with controls who do not have the outcome. The process of comparison aims at identifying characteristics that are different in persons who have the problem or outcome of interest compared with persons who do not have the problem or outcome. By comparing these two groups, we may be able to detect differences that lead to the identification of factors associated with the detrimental outcome.

The comparison group that does not have the outcome of interest is used as a control or reference group. The control group provides an estimate of the frequency of the various characteristics being tested as associated with the outcome of interest. Although randomized clinical trials have provided the best approach for evaluating the efficacy of mammographic screening in preventing deaths from breast cancer, if we need to evaluate the same procedure using the case-control method, our cases may be persons dying from breast cancer, while our controls will be women from the same population, of similar age, who do not have the outcome of death from breast cancer. The controls will provide the frequency of mammography in the community if the procedure had no impact on death from breast cancer. To determine whether the resurgence of measles in a community is the result of a failure of the vaccination program in this population, the comparison group to our cases of measles will be persons who do not have measles and are comparable to the cases as to certain characteristics, such as age. Thus, to establish comparability between cases and controls, we want to select a comparison group from the same population as the cases. Comparability also will ensure that cases and controls are similar with regard to important variables that will affect the relation between the outcome and exposure. The control group will provide us with an estimate of the frequency of mammographic screening or measles vaccination in the same population. The case-control method, in addition, will allow us to compare the two groups as to the frequency of other possible determinants. For example, in addition to mammographic screening, it would be possible to investigate other determinants of death from breast cancer, including attributes of medical care, risk factors for the incidence of breast cancer, etc.

Measuring exposure

We may use a number of approaches to collect data about the various characteristics of cases and controls. These include interviews, questionnaires, and various forms of previously recorded information. Major issues with collecting such data include potential problems of validity and reliability, as well as misclassification. In our previous example of a case-control study of vaccination and measles, it is possible to collect data about the vaccination status of the study population by interviewing the subjects or some proxy respondents, but it is also possible to collect detailed data about vaccination status from medical records. The records, in this case, also may provide us with data about the source and batch of vaccine, the process of vaccination, etc. However, the personal interview allows us to collect additional information about the cases and controls that is not recorded and that may represent important determinants or confounders of the relation between vaccination and outcome of measles, for example, coverage and access to medical care, changes in sources of medical care, education of parents, and religious and cultural differentials. A number of case-control studies incorporate laboratory measurements of various biologic parameters to supplement information from interviews and medical records.

Estimating risk

In epidemiology, we ascertain the risk of disease for various exposures by estimating two measures: relative and attributable risks. The relative risk is based on a ratio of two incidence rates, that is, the incidence of the disease in the exposed to the incidence in the nonexposed. Since in a case-control study it is not possible to calculate incidence rates, the odds ratio provides an alternative measure of risk. In particular, for a situation where the outcome is rare, we can estimate the relative risk by calculating the odds ratio. Although the odds ratio is not based on two incidence rates, it provides a measure of association between the outcome and the exposure.

In addition to a comparison of the frequency of exposure in the case and control groups, the case-control method allows us to calculate two odds of exposure: the odds of cases being exposed compared with the odds of controls for the same exposure. Odds represent the ratio of two frequencies. The ratio of the odds in the cases over the odds in the controls is the odds ratio. For example, the odds of exposure to vaccines in the cases of measles are compared with the odds of vaccination in the controls. If vaccination is protective for measles, then the odds of vaccine exposure in the cases of measles will be smaller than those in the controls and the odds ratio will be less than 1.

As seen in Table 8-2, the odds ratio is expressed as a ratio of the product of the number exposed in the cases and the number nonexposed in the controls to the product of the number nonexposed in the cases and the number exposed in the controls. Thus, if our hypothesis states that aspirin causes Reye's syndrome in children, the odds ratio will have as a numerator the product of the frequency of our cases with Reye's syndrome who have used aspirin and the frequency of controls who have not used aspirin and our denominator will be the product of the frequency of cases who have not used aspirin and the frequency of controls who have used aspirin. If the numerator is larger than the denominator, we may confirm our hypothesis that there is an association between Reye's syndrome and aspirin intake.

Attributable risk assesses the importance of a particular factor explaining the load of the disease or adverse outcome in the community. An attributable risk of 70% for aspirin in Reye's syndrome means that 70% of cases in that particular community could be explained by aspirin intake. This measure may differ between communities since, as a measure, it is dependent on the frequency of exposure in the community.

Thus, for each of the suspected determinants of the outcome, the case-control method allows us to study the relative importance of these factors. Depression and arthritis are two known causes of disability. The case-control method allows us to estimate the relative importance of these as determinants of disability in general, by estimating the odds ratios, and for the population under consideration, it permits the calculation of specific attributable risks for arthritis and depression.

In addition to the individual effect of the various characteristics, the case-control method allows us to assess whether there is any interaction between these various factors. Thus, using the same example as above, a possible interaction between antecedent depression and arthritis as determinants of disability has been studied (H. K. Armenian et al., unpublished observation).

Table 8-2. Estimation of odds ratios

	Cases	*Controls*
Exposed	A	B
Nonexposed	C	D

$$Odds\ ratio = \frac{A/C}{B/D} = \frac{AD}{BC}$$

A method for evaluation

A number of interventions have been evaluated using the case-control method. These investigations have included evaluations of vaccine efficacy and vaccination effectiveness, in particular with BCG vaccines in tuberculosis; assessments of screening programs for cervical, breast, and colon cancers; evaluations of medical therapies; and a number of programmatic activities in the community. In the absence of the possibility of setting up randomized clinical trials to evaluate efficacy and in situations where an intervention is already widely utilized in the community, the case-control method may present a good and efficient alternative for the evaluation of interventions.

The case-control method is efficient for generating an appropriate information base for policy decisions. The method is used for decision-making in a number of situations of policy formulation.

The rest of this chapter addresses the needs of health professionals at two levels of application of the case-control method. The first of these involves the understanding and evaluation of reported and published case-control studies. The second involves guidelines about the design and implementation of case-control studies within the framework of health services management and evaluation.

Assessing Published Case-Control Studies

The quality of published case-control studies is quite variable. Despite the close scrutiny that most journals apply to the review of what is published, readers sometimes encounter reports that have methodological problems. Some of these problems are situational in that what is presented is the best possible study under difficult circumstances and limited resources. However, for a number of these problems, there may be alternative solutions. It is up to the reader to make a judgment as to the validity of the approaches used and the inferences made on the basis of the data presented. An informed and educated reader will avoid costly decisions based on inappropriate information.

Table 8-3 lists eight questions that should be asked when reviewing a reported case-control study. This list encourages us to think of alternative approaches in dealing with issues of design in case-control studies. Following are two case studies of case-control reports, to illustrate the process of evaluation of published reports.

Case study 1

Abstract: Over 13 million people in the United States wear soft contact lenses for refractive correction. Ulcerative keratitis is considered the most serious adverse effect of the use of contact lenses. We performed a case-control study with 86 case patients, estimating separately for hospital-based ($n = 61$) and population-based ($n = 410$) controls the relative risk of ulcerative keratitis among users of extended-wear as compared with daily wear soft contact lenses.

The relative risk of ulcerative keratitis for extended-wear as compared with daily-wear lenses among the population-based controls was 3.90 (95 percent confidence interval, 2.35 to 6.48) and among the hospital-based controls, eight percent of those with extended-wear lenses used them only during the day, and 11 percent of those with daily-wear lenses occasionally wore them overnight. When lens wearers were distinguished according to their overnight use of lenses, the users of extended-wear lenses who wore them overnight had a risk 10 to 15 times as great as the users of daily-wear lenses who did not, and the users of daily-wear lenses who sometimes wore them overnight had 9 times the risk of the users of such lenses who did not. For the users of extended-wear lenses, the risk of ulcerative keratitis was incrementally related to the extent of overnight wear. A reduction in risk associated with more frequent attention to lens hygiene was almost significant.

We conclude that the soft contact lenses worn overnight carry a significantly greater risk for ulcerative keratitis than soft lenses worn only during the day (Schein et al., 1989).

1. How is the problem defined?

[It is estimated that] over 13 million people in the United States wear soft contact lenses. [A number of] adverse effects have been reported with all types of lenses, [and] the most serious complication—ulcerative keratitis—has been linked most closely to the use of soft lenses. [The authors aimed at determining] the relative risk of ulcerative keratitis in those who use cosmetic, extended-wear soft contact lenses as compared with those who use cosmetic, daily-wear soft contact lenses (Schein et al., 1989).

The problem statement in the introduction of this paper provides a clear perspective of the public health importance of the issue and delineates the problem

Table 8-3. Questions for assessment of case-control studies

1. Is there a clear definition of the problem under consideration?
2. Is the definition of cases consistent with the definition of the problem?
3. Are the controls selected from the same base population as the cases?
4. How valid is the measurement of the exposure(s) under consideration?
5. Is the process of selecting the cases and controls independent of the approach used to get information about exposure?
6. Has the analysis considered the potential role of alternative explanations to the association under investigation (confounding)?
7. Are there potential interactions between the various factors the authors have studied?
8. What is the information value of the published report with respect to the decision process in health services?

geographically to the United States and to the population of users of extended-wear soft contact lenses worn for cosmetic purposes. Although broader generalizations may be of interest, this study does not aim, for example, at studying all causes of keratitis.

2. Is the definition of cases consistent with the definition of the problem?

> Ninety-nine patients with ulcerative keratitis associated with the use of soft contact lenses for cosmetic purposes were enrolled prospectively between November 1986 and November 1987 from six university ophthalmologic centers across the United States. . . . Eligible case patients were 12 years of age or older, spoke English or Spanish, wore cosmetic soft lenses . . . and underwent verification of their case status by corneal specialists from the participating centers. Patients who wore hard or rigid gas-permeable lenses were excluded, as were patients who wore soft lenses for aphakia or therapeutic reasons (Schein et al., 1989).

Having limited the problem to the population of cosmetic users of soft contact lenses, the authors define their cases very appropriately within the same population. Although one may raise questions of the representativeness of these cases from six specialized centers across the United States, the authors probably were more concerned with the diagnostic validity of the cases under consideration.

3. Are the controls selected from the same population as the cases?

> Two control groups were enrolled: hospital-based controls—people who wore soft contact lenses and who presented to the eye centers for acute conditions unrelated to lens use—and population-based controls who wore soft contact lenses for cosmetic purposes and were identified by random-digit dialing in a telephone survey. . . . A hospital-based control was defined as a wearer of cosmetic soft contact lenses, 12 years of age or older and speaking English or Spanish. . . . Hospital-based controls were recruited from the same clinical sources as the case patients. [In identifying population-based controls,] for each case patient, matched households were selected by random-digit dialing based on the area code and first four digits of the case patient's home telephone number (Schein et al., 1989).

The investigators have tried to make the cases and controls comparable based on a number of characteristics. The hospital-based controls provide such comparability since they are identified from the same group of patients who are users of soft contact lenses for cosmetic purposes only. Random-digit dialing identifies a second group of controls that is more representative of the base population under study and allows generalization of the findings beyond the patients studied from the hospitals.

4. How valid is the measurement of the exposure(s) under consideration?

> [A] 20-minute interview was conducted with the use of a computer-assisted telephone interviewing system. The interview had five major sections. The first

confirmed eligibility and determined the type of lens worn. The second recorded the general medical and ophthalmic history. The third examined lens use and care, including 23 measures of the four tasks of basic hygiene. . . . The fourth and fifth sections gathered information on previous use of lenses, demographic characteristics, and instructions received. . . . Specific lens-care habits were investigated for the two-month period before the first hospital visit of the case patients and the hospital-based controls and for the two months before the population-based controls were interviewed by telephone (Schein et al., 1989).

The main exposures that concern the investigators in this study relate to the different patterns of use of the contact lenses and to the hygienic procedures used by the study subjects. The interview generates an extensive data base on a number of factors relevant to the problem under investigation. As per the description of the authors, cases and controls were interviewed using the same methods. Thus, there is a very strong likelihood that the data obtained have a high level of reliability. However, with the use of two control groups, one may have two estimates of risk since the exposure patterns may be different. If differences between the control groups arise, interpretation of such differences may shed new light on the observations. In this report, the authors do not present any information about the validity of the data collected using this particular interview technique. Further, potential biases of information in case-control studies involve misclassification of exposure due to shortcomings of interview procedures and interviewee response. From the description of the methods in this paper, we are not able to assess adequately the validity of the exposure information.

> *5. Is the process of selecting the cases and controls independent from the approach used to get information about exposure?*

Could the way in which the cases and controls were selected for this study influence the validity and reliability of the information from the study subjects? For example, would the interviewing process permit a more rigorous effort with the cases compared with the controls in the collection of data about potentially adverse practices? Is there a possibility that, in the selection of the study subjects, more cases were identified selectively from patients with adverse practices than controls? From a review of the methods used for the selection of cases and controls and the high level of comparability of the procedures used, it is unlikely that such a selection bias could have occurred in this study. The use of two control groups, one of which is population-based and randomly identified, gives further credence to the findings of the study. Consistency of findings in the analysis, using the two control groups separately, supports this idea.

> *6. Has the analysis considered the potential role of alternative explanations to the association under investigation?*

Statistical analyses were conducted with the use of unconditional logistic-regression models adjusted for the variables used in matching. Analyses were performed in parallel, once to compare case patients with hospital-based controls and a second time to compare case patients with population-based controls. Since hospital-based controls were matched with case patients on the basis of center and gender, analyses that compared the two groups included terms for center, sex, and the interaction between them (Schein et al., 1989).

The alternative explanations considered by the authors include the potential for confounding for a number of variables. Thus, during the design phase of the study, they established a high level of comparability of cases and controls, particularly with regard to age, gender, center or location, and access to health services. These are factors that could act as potential confounders. Each of these variables could give us an association between adverse practices and ulcerative keratitis if not adjusted for or matched. Hence, in addition to design maneuvers, the investigators conducted a number of adjustments and confirmed their findings following these analyses.

> *7. Are there potential interactions between various factors that the authors have studied?*

Table 2 (Schein et al., 1989) of the paper presents data that can be used to calculate the interaction between two variables: lens type and overnight use. Considering daily wear lenses in those with no overnight use as the lowest risk group of 1.00, extended wear lenses with no overnight use had a relative risk estimate of about 2.6, daily wear lenses with overnight use had a risk estimate of about 9.3, and the combined daily wear group with overnight use and extended wear lenses had a relative risk estimate of about 12.5.

These relative risk estimates could form the basis of estimating a weak additive interaction between these two variables. The report does not elaborate on any further analysis of more complex models of interaction.

> *8. What is the information value of the published report with respect to the decision process in health services?*

> For the users of extended-wear lenses, the risk of ulcerative keratitis was incrementally related to the extent of overnight wear. A reduction in risk associated with more frequent attention to lens hygiene was almost significant. . . . We conclude that soft contact lenses worn overnight carry a significantly greater risk for ulcerative keratitis than soft lenses worn only during the day. . . . Although our data strongly indicated that the overnight use of soft lenses was the principal risk factor for ulcerative keratitis, the part that lens care can play in this risk and in future efforts to lessen it deserves mention (Schein et al., 1989).

The information generated by this investigation is directly applicable at the clinical level as well as within the framework of public health action. This particular case-control study has made our knowledge of ulcerative keratitis in contact lens users more specific and useful for prevention. This information allows us to identify the subgroup that needs to be targeted for preventive action, and it gives us a focus for intervention.

This investigation handles a number of important issues in case-control studies. It deals with a problem within a well-defined target population. It uses two different control groups to study the problem. The use of two control groups allows the authors to address some potential problems with selection and information biases. The investigators used random-digit dialing for identifying one of their control groups, as well as interviewing controls. Their concern with confounding is addressed at both the design and analysis phases of the study. The analysis also tries to identify potential interactions between the variables of interest.

Case study 2

Abstract

Objective—To investigate the relation between suboptimal intrapartum obstetric care and cerebral palsy or death.

Design—Case-control study.

Setting—Oxford Regional Health Authority.

Subjects—141 babies who subsequently developed cerebral palsy and 62 who died intrapartum or neonatally, 1984–7. All subjects were born at term of singleton pregnancies and had no congenital anomaly. Two controls, matched for place and time of birth, were selected for each index case.

Main outcome measures—Adverse antenatal factors and suboptimal intrapartum care (by using predefined criteria).

Results—Failure to respond to signs of severe fetal distress was more common in cases of cerebral palsy (odds ratio 4.5; 95% confidence interval 2.4 to 8.4) and in cases of death (26.1; 6.2 to 109.7) than among controls. This association persisted even after adjustment for increased incidence of a complicated obstetric history in cases of cerebral palsy. Neonatal encephalopathy is regarded as the best clinical indicator of birth asphyxia; only two thirds (23/33) of the children with cerebral palsy in whom there had been a suboptimal response to fetal distress, however, had evidence of neonatal encephalopathy; these 23 formed 6.8% of all children with cerebral palsy born to residents of the region in the four years studied.

Conclusion—There is an association between quality of intrapartum care and death. The findings also suggest an association between suboptimal care and cerebral palsy, but this seems to have a role in only a small proportion of all cases of cerebral palsy. The contribution of adverse antenatal factors in the origin of cerebral palsy needs further study (Gaffney et al., 1994).

1. How is the problem defined?

The relation between the quality of care which is given to a mother during labor and delivery and the death of her baby or cerebral palsy in her surviving child is a continuing source of debate involving obstetricians, pediatricians, parents, and

> lawyers. . . . [W]e tested the null hypothesis that compared with controls, cases of cerebral palsy among singleton babies born at term without congenital anomaly are not more likely to have been preceded by intrapartum care defined by preset criteria and considered by clinical consensus to be suboptimal. [The authors highlight the possibility that factors antedating the intrapartum period may be responsible for cerebral palsy and death.] Further, it is possible that signs of fetal distress in babies who later manifest cerebral palsy may reflect previous antenatal factors rather than an acute intrapartum hypoxic event (Gaffney et al., 1994).

Although the authors state clearly the research problem they are tackling, they do not provide a statement of the size of the public health problem involved. Such a statement is needed to highlight the epidemiologic dimensions of the problem. However, the authors point to the relatively complex nature of the problem and, as such, limit their study to a subgroup of the case population, to deal partially with this complex issue.

2. Is the definition of the cases consistent with the definition of the problem?

> *Cerebral palsy*—Children with cerebral palsy born in 1984–7 who were singleton deliveries, born at 37 weeks' gestation or more, and who had no congenital anomaly or postnatal cause were identified from the Oxford region register of early childhood impairments. The definition of cerebral palsy used by the register is that of a permanent impairment of voluntary movement or posture presumed to be due to permanent damage to the immature brain. . . .
> *Deaths*—Intrapartum stillbirths and deaths occurring after birth among babies born at 37 weeks' gestation and with no major congenital anomaly and with no evidence of severe infection were identified from copies of death certificates (previously obtained by the Oxford region register of early childhood impairment) and from the records of each maternity unit (Gaffney et al., 1994).

The authors are dealing with two outcomes: cerebral palsy and death. Both of these outcomes are to be studied in terms of their relation to intrapartum care. To minimize the possibility of some cases being related to factors preceding the intrapartum period, they have eliminated from their case groups

> cases of cerebral palsy children who were born preterm or of a multiple pregnancy and those with a known congenital anomaly. In this way we anticipated that the cases of cerebral palsy remaining would include those most likely to be associated with suboptimal intrapartum care—that is, obstetrically preventable (Gaffney et al., 1994).

Similarly, the authors have excluded from their cases deaths occurring before 37 weeks of gestation and deaths with evidence of congenital anomaly or severe infection. Thus, by using such a case definition, the study is limited to the question of whether cerebral palsy and death in children are potentially preventable by intrapartum care. The selection of cases is community-based and probably representative of all such cases in the Oxford region.

3. Are the controls selected from the same population as the cases?

> Two controls for each case were selected by identifying in each hospital delivery book the two babies born immediately before the index case. Only singleton babies born at 37 weeks' gestation or after and with no major congenital anomaly were included. Controls were drawn from all 10 of the hospitals in the region that provide obstetric care (Gaffney et al., 1994).

In selecting their controls, the investigators have used the same criteria as for the cases ($\geq$37 weeks of gestation, absence of congenital malformations). Considering that the vast majority of the deliveries are performed within hospitals, the controls are selected from the 10 area hospitals that provide obstetric care.

4. How valid is the measurement of the exposure(s) under consideration?

> [In a review with] every obstetrician in the region, agreement could not be reached on which items should be included in the assessment of antenatal care, but after a lot of discussion a consensus was reached on the criteria for suboptimal care. The criteria for suboptimal resuscitation after delivery were based on the recommendations of the Royal College of Obstetricians and Gynecologists. . . . A decision was made that there had been a suboptimal response to signs of intrapartum fetal distress [when these criteria were not met] (Gaffney et al., 1994).

Since the authors of this study are evaluating the effect of intrapartum care, the latter is the exposure that they need to measure. There are many problems with defining what constitutes adequate quality of care in such a clinical situation. The approach used is that of developing a consensus between the practitioners involved with the care of this patient population. The consensus is based on criteria that have been accepted by professional groups or for similar research. It is important to note that these criteria are defined prior to the initiation of the study and that the authors strive to produce objective measures of what may be considered appropriate care.

5. Is the process of selecting the cases and controls independent of the approach used to get information about exposure?

> The obstetric notes of mothers included in the study were obtained. All information about the outcome of the baby was masked by a researcher who did not participate in the review of the notes; and the notes were reviewed by a researcher blind to the neonatal condition and the child's outcome. . . . A second observer (a consultant obstetrician), also blind to the outcome of the baby and using the same criteria, then made an independent assessment of the quality of intrapartum care. When there was disagreement between the two observers a

third person was asked to act as arbiter. This was rarely necessary as the criteria were so precise. . . . Finally, information from the pediatric notes was abstracted, including the condition at delivery and evidence of neonatal encephalopathy (Gaffney et al., 1994).

The initial identification of cases and controls was based on special registers, while the information about obstetric care and covariates was collected from chart reviews. As noted above, the authors have made a special effort to keep the process of outcome assessment independent of the process of collecting information about the hypothesized determinants of the outcome, that is, the characteristics of the obstetric care. Blinding of the record review was one approach used by the authors. The use of pediatric notes as another independent source of outcome assessment (also by a blinded observer) gives further credence to the independence of the two processes.

6. Has the analysis considered the potential role of alternative explanations to the association under investigation?

Analysis entailed the comparison of two case series, cerebral palsy and death, with controls matched for hospital and time of birth. The relative odds for particular antenatal and intrapartum characteristics and the likelihood of the presence of these characteristics were estimated by using only matched sets. . . . The relative odds were based only on discordant sets—that is, sets in which the presence or absence of the characteristics differed between the cases and controls. . . . The odds ratio is an estimate of the odds of suboptimal care among cases relative to the odds of suboptimal care among controls. . . . Further analysis was performed to examine the confounding effect of having had a complicated antenatal history on the association of cerebral palsy and quality of care (Gaffney et al., 1994).

The alternative explanations considered by the authors include potential sources of bias that have been dealt with at the design phase of the study (as discussed in question 5 above) and confounding by a number of factors that may affect the outcome of the pregnancy and may be related to the type of intrapartum care received by the mother, such as complicated antenatal history. In addition to matching, the authors made adjustments to study the potential role of various suspected confounders.

7. What is the information value of the published paper with respect to the decision process in health services?

Mothers of term, singleton, non-malformed babies who die or who later have a cerebral palsy have an increased risk of a complicated antenatal course. They also have an increased risk of having signs of intrapartum fetal distress and a suboptimal response to this distress. . . . [These are some of the conclusions of the authors. In their final paragraph, they emphasize the following.] Our findings support, however, the view that birth events, avoidable or unavoidable, are contributing factors in only a few cases of cerebral palsy. Even among this highly selected group of term singleton, non-malformed cases of cerebral palsy over two thirds had no signs of intrapartum distress. The challenge for the clinician is the small group of children with cerebral palsy with apparently potentially avoidable intrapartum hypoxia; the challenge for researchers is to determine much more precisely the interrelations of chronic intrauterine hypoxia and other antenatal events, neonatal encephalopathy, and cerebral palsy (Gaffney et al., 1994).

The authors present in a separate table the clinical implications of their findings. The broader policy implications for this case-control study are not addressed in the discussion.

This study presents a rare feature in case-control studies in that it assesses the effect of care on two outcomes. Thus, the use of two case groups allows the authors to do ''two case-control studies in one.'' Considering the complex nature of the different elements involved in intrapartum care, the case-control study is appropriate for delineating the contribution of the various components of such care to the outcomes of interest.

Guidelines for Designing a Case-Control Study

There are no ''gold standards'' for case-control studies. There are problems that need to be addressed. Being sensitive about these problems improves our ability to design and assess these studies. Following are some general guidelines for designing case-control studies.

1. Define clearly the problem under consideration and the reference population in which the problem will be examined. This step will affect everything else. Case-control studies may be exploratory or may be designed to test a specific hypothesis. The problem definition will dictate case definition and guide case and control selection.
2. Decide the type and selection process of controls. This step will affect validity and generalizability.
3. Develop a process of data collection that depends on instruments of high-level validity and reliability. In ascertaining potential sources of biases, be careful that the process of case and control selection is independent of the approach used for data collection about the particular factor(s) under consideration.
4. Decide what are confounders for the particular study and the approach to be used in dealing with them. There are alternative approaches to taking care of confounding. Matching will establish comparability as to the confounders in the design phase of the study. Establishing comparability is also dictated by having cases and controls from the same reference popula-

tion. (In an evaluation of interventions, it is often important to assess the comparability of the different exposure groups relative to confounders that relate the intervention to the outcome. Such an assessment will address the issue of whether the exposed and the nonexposed groups came from the same population and had similar opportunities for exposure to the intervention. The latter will help us in our inferences as to considerations of efficacy and effectiveness. If the exposed and nonexposed groups are similar as to all known and potential confounders, then the study could be one of efficacy.)

5. Following are other practical guidelines that will improve the efficiency of case-control studies:
   • Why consider a case-control design for this problem rather than an alternative?
   • What is the additional information value of the case-control study?
   • What is unique or what is the special advantage of the case-control method in addressing this problem or hypothesis?

These guidelines are to be used with an understanding that every study has its own set of problems and may need a different set of solutions. The third case study uses these guidelines in designing a case-control study on the impact of primary care on subsequent hospitalization.

Case study 3

The rising cost of medical care has forced decision-makers to evaluate existing methods of care and to consider potentially more cost-effective alternatives. Considering that hospitalization is the single most expensive component of the medical care bill, approaches that decrease hospitalization rates are of high interest to decision-makers. A number of initiatives have focused on improving primary medical care as a way of reducing health care costs. In addition to its effect as a measure of cost containment, primary medical care potentially could reduce hospitalization by preventing illness or its serious manifestations.

The state of B has a population of 350,000 and a system of health care based on a large network of primary health care centers. Traditionally, the system was based on hospital care and hospital outpatient facilities serving as the main source of primary care for the population. The large investment by the government of B to build a network of primary health care centers was justified by planners as a method of cost containment. The minister of health of the state of B is interested in testing this assumption and would like to know whether the use of primary care facilities would prevent expensive hospitalization. The minister is requesting an investigation that would test the idea and would provide answers within the next 3 months.

Problem and case definition. Consider that you are asked to conduct this investigation. What is your formulation of the problem or the hypothesis that you are asked to test? On the basis of your formulation of the hypothesis, could you define your cases ?

The research problem that we need to deal with is whether use of primary care facilities decreases hospitalization. Our definition of the problem will thus mandate the selection of cases as persons who are hospitalized, if we want to pursue the case-control method of investigation. (At this stage, you may like to review the advantages and disadvantages of the case-control method.) The reasons for using the case-control method in conducting this particular investigation include efficiency and informativeness. We need to provide answers to the minister of health within 3 months, and we can conduct our study with a limited study population. Also, we may be able to incorporate in our study a large number of persons with the outcome (hospitalization). We may also be able to inquire in our data collection phase about a number of variables and processes within the primary care system that may affect hospitalization.

Selection of controls. The controls represent the subgroup of our population who do not have the outcome under investigation. What are some alternative approaches of selecting controls?

Following are some options for control groups that may be used in this investigation:

1. Neighbors of hospitalized cases
2. Other patients from the same clinic as the cases
3. The general population, selected by random digit dialing
4. Randomly selected visitors, who are in the hospital as a social obligation

Although we can add a few more options to the selection of controls, our scrutiny of the listed options indicates that each of the proposed control groups highlights a different strategy in identifying the determinant(s) of hospitalization. Thus, option 1 selects the controls from the same population and geographic subgroup as the cases and assumes that the determinant(s) for hospitalization and primary care use vary by neighborhood of residence. Selecting controls from other patients in the same clinic, as in option 2, ensures that the controls have some opportunity of use of the primary care system; however, these controls will not include any person who has not used the primary care facilities. Such a control group will overestimate the effect of primary care in preventing hospitalization. Random digit dialing, as listed in option 3, introduces a random process in the selection of our controls and, thus, may give us a representative comparison group from the population; however, such a selection of controls is limited by ownership of telephones and the end product may not be as representative of the general population as we may expect. The extensive use of answering machines and cellular telephones and other future changes of communication technologies may adversely affect the selection of controls by random digit dialing by limiting access to potential controls or further selecting a subgroup of the target population. Visitors to hospital patients have been used in a few studies as a source of controls. Such controls provide a nondiseased comparison group that may be representative of the general population. However, such a control group is useful mainly in a cultural environment where visiting hospital patients is a strong social obligation and, thus, a large sector of the general population makes social visits to hospitals (Armenian et al., 1988). It is also important that the factor under consideration (i.e., use of primary care facilities) does not influence the ability of individuals to be visitors to hospital patients.

The optimal decision may be to select more than one type of control group. Using more than one type of control group may allow us to test the hypothesis in more ways than one. Agreement in the results using the different control groups separately strengthens our confidence in the findings. However, if the results from the two control groups are discrepant, then interpreting such discrepancies by taking into consideration the different characteristics of the control groups will be a very useful process in our effort to elucidate the underlying determinants of the problem under study.

Data collection. The process of data collection is determined by the hypotheses that are formulated. Considering that we are dealing with a number of options that could explain hospitalization, what are the various elements of information that we are interested in collecting about the cases and controls?

To develop a list of possible hypotheses, we may use the following maneuvers:

1. Review of the literature
2. Discussion with experts
3. Review of a subgroup of cases

Having considered a number of hypotheses, we must make decisions about the sources of data to be used, the limitations of these sources, the possibility of using more than one alternative data source for the same information, etc. In our particular study, we will need to collect data about the use of health centers by both cases and controls, most probably by a review of medical records, but we also will need to collect information on the types and severity of morbidity, as well as data about the content of the care these individuals received within the primary care system.

Confounders. Decisions about how to deal with alternative interpretations in case-control studies are made at both the design and the analysis phases. Delimiting the cases and controls, matching, stratification, and adjustment are some of the approaches used to deal with confounding. Define for the stated hypothesis the potential confounders and make decisions as to your preferred process of dealing with these confounders.

A number of factors may need to be considered as confounders in this study. Demographic characteristics, such as age and sex, are probably related to both hospitalization and the use of primary care facilities. Thus, we will need to establish comparability as to age and gender between the cases and controls. Individual or frequency matching on age and gender is one approach. In addition to demographic characteristics, there are other covariates, as illustrated in the previous section. Thus, the severity and nature of illness are important determinants of use of the primary health center, as is hospitalization. We may decide, for example, to stratify our analysis by some indicator of severity. We may also decide that we will adjust for these potential confounders at the analysis phase of the study.

Interpretation. Before data collection, it is very useful to develop a number of blank tables with the variables under consideration and to list the various possible directions in which the data may be distributed. Within the current proposed project, one such dummy table will have case-control status in the columns and the number of clinic visits in the rows. We may list all possible interpretations if there were no difference in the number of visits between the cases and controls, if the cases had a higher number of visits than the controls, or if the results were as expected by the study hypothesis. Such an approach will allow us to identify deficiencies in the data being collected, especially if such a theoretical review is done prior to the implementation phase of the study. It will be a worthwhile exercise to prepare three such dummy tables and to interpret the various projected options in the findings.

Future Applications

As discussed previously, the case-control method has been used for a large number of problem-solving situations. As the number of new uses for such studies has increased, different sets of methodological issues have emerged.

The revolution in information technology and the resulting explosive growth in the number of large data bases will provide opportunities for epidemiologists to conduct a large number of investigations on data that are readily available. The introduction of new systems for delivering health services will encourage closer scrutiny of the costs and benefits of interventions and providers. The need for better and more efficient instruments of evaluation will prompt more extensive use of the case-control method. This will help to enhance the integration of epidemiologic methods into the decision-making process at both policy and operational levels.

Possible future developments in the use of the case-control method include the following, adapted from Armenian and Gordis (1994).

Ongoing surveillance and analysis

Some of the established information systems, including epidemiologic surveillance programs, may apply a sequential approach in analyzing data on an ongoing basis using the case-control method. With such an approach, as specific outcomes are reported to the information system, data also will be collected routinely from appropriate controls, and a case-control analysis can be conducted whenever there are enough cases to provide adequate statistical power to the study. Thus, health information systems may become more analytic in their approaches, and they may help to identify leads to etiology and for further investigation. Case-control analyses likely will be an increasingly important part of the routine reports prepared by these information systems.

Rapid case-control analyses

With electronic linkages between available data bases and packaged programs, it will be possible to conduct case-control analyses in a very rapid manner. Thus, the case-control method will become a more efficient approach to problem-solving in epidemiology and more valuable in providing timely answers to critical questions.

Conclusions

Some of the lessons of this chapter include the following:

1. Problem definition and its linkage to the definition of cases are important. A well-circumscribed and -delineated problem is critical to case definition.
2. The case definition in turn will determine our process of control selection.
3. To avoid information and selection biases, we must keep the process of selection of cases and controls independent of the process of data collection about exposures.
4. We may use a number of alternative approaches in dealing with confounding.
5. All case-control studies need to investigate the possibility of interaction between the various factors of interest.

6. Every projected study needs to assess the information value of the data collection effort prior to its implementation. What will be the policy implications of the proposed study?

References

Armenian, H. K., and L. Gordis. 1994. Future perspectives. *Epidemiol. Rev.*, 16:163–164.

Armenian, H. K., N. G. Lakkis, A. M. Sibai, et al. 1988. Hospital visitors as controls. *Am. J. Epidemiol.*, 127:404–406.

Armenian, H. K. and D. E. Lilienfeld. 1994. Overview and historical perspective. *Epidemiol Rev.*, 16:1–5.

Brook, R. H., J. E. Ware, W. H. Rogers, et al. 1983. Does free care improve adults' health? Results of a randomized controlled trial. *N. Engl. J. Med.*, 309:1426–1434.

Comstock, G. W. 1994. Evaluating vaccination effectiveness and vaccine efficacy by means of case-control studies. *Epidemiol. Rev.*, 16:77–89.

Gaffney, G., S. Sellers, V. Flavell, et al. 1994. Case-control study of intrapartum care, cerebral palsy, and perinatal death. *BMJ*, 308:743–750.

Greenland, S., E. Watson, and R. R. Neutra. 1981. The case-control method in medical care evaluation. *Med. Care*, 19:872–878.

Newhouse, J. P. 1974. A design for a health insurance experiment. *Inquiry*, 11:5–27.

Schein, O. D., R. J. Glynn, E. C. Poggio, et al. 1989. The relative risk of ulcerative keratitis among users of daily-wear and extended wear soft contact lenses: a case-control study. *N. Engl. J. Med.*, 321:773–778.

Selby, J. V. 1994. Case-control evaluation of treatment and program efficacy. *Epidemiol. Rev.*, 16:90–101.

CHAPTER 9

Randomized Controlled Trials in Health Services Research

SAM SHAPIRO

The randomized controlled trial (RCT) is recognized as the most rigorous method available for testing hypotheses in the health care field. It is a longitudinal, prospective method in which a population or defined set of subjects is randomly allocated into subgroups ''to receive or not to receive an experimental preventive or therapeutic procedure, maneuver, or intervention'' (Last, 1988, p. 110). The objective is to determine the efficacy or effectiveness of the intervention through the comparison of a defined outcome in an experimental group and a control group.

The strength of the RCT was first demonstrated by Sir Bradford Hill in the Streptomycin in Tuberculosis Trials (1948). Many other trials have been conducted since then. In the United States, the RCT has been applied to a wide variety of problems, including treating patients with antihypertensive agents (Freis, 1967), testing the efficacy of intervening on risk factors for coronary heart disease (Multiple Risk Factor Intervention Trial Group, 1977), determining the role of lumpectomy for breast cancer treatment (Fisher and Redmond, 1992), and analyzing the effect on costs of substituting community care for nursing home care for the frail elderly (Kemper, 1988). Two RCTs are taken up later as case examples.

An essential component of all of these studies has been adherence to the principle of randomization. Statistical studies typically involve comparisons between subgroups, and confidence in the results is indicated by the degree to which we are able to control for confounding variables (i.e., the effect of an exposure on risk is distorted because of its association with other factors that influence the outcome). The achievement of absolute control, however, is most often illusory in observational studies. In an RCT, the goals are to achieve equality between study and control groups in all characteristics at the start of the study, to avoid the problem of confounding, and to maintain equality between the two groups throughout the study except for the intervention being tested.

This chapter probes into key elements of the RCT; examines its strengths in deciding whether, for example, a change advocated in health care practices should be adopted; considers the design and conduct of an RCT; and weighs the issues that arise in generalizing the results. This is accomplished first by specifying a set of questions fundamental to understanding the RCT, then by discussing them. Case studies drawn from published reports are used to illustrate the points made. A series of questions is raised at the end of each case study based on the material presented. These questions should stimulate the reader to think about more general issues affecting the choice and conduct of studies.

- Is there a well-formulated hypothesis?
- What are the ethical issues that affect the conduct of an RCT?
- What is the function of randomization in an RCT? How does randomization theoretically control for bias and confounding variables?
- What methods of randomization are available to achieve comparability between intervention and control groups?
- What is the role of stratification in selecting samples for the intervention and control groups?
- How does an RCT based on volunteers differ from an RCT based on samples from a defined universe?
- What is meant by contamination ("once randomized, always randomized")? How are crossovers and drop-outs defined in an RCT? How are they handled analytically?
- How certain should we be that the sample is large enough to detect a prespecified effect attributable to the intervention?
- How long should the experiment run?
- How are the results of an RCT interpreted? What are the limitations on generalizability of results. What are the requirements for broadening generalizability?

Major Issues in an RCT

The need for well-formulated hypotheses

The hypothesis for an RCT must be sharply formulated, with the outcome open to question. Without conflicting views, it would be difficult and, in many instances, impossible to initiate an RCT. The untested procedure should have laboratory results, exploratory studies, or a strong theoretic justification for expecting success in the experiment.

For example, low birth weight infants are at increased risk for developmental delay and for a variety of medical complications compared with their normal birth weight counterparts. They tend to have lower scores on tests of cognitive functioning, are more prone to difficulties in behavioral adjustment, and are at risk for having learning problems and poor academic achievements. Further, the likelihood of adverse development and scholastic outcomes is greater in the face of socioeconomic disadvantage.

Interest in the future health and welfare of children at risk for poor developmental outcome has focused attention on the potential of interventions in changing the situation among low birth weight, premature infants. Prior RCTs had encouraged the likelihood of change, but skepticism existed, particularly about what could be achieved among low birth weight infants. This led to an RCT to test the hypothesis that structured day care starting at age 12 months and family support services starting at birth would reduce developmental, behavioral, and health problems among low birth weight, premature infants by the age of 3 years (A Multisite Randomized Trial, 1990).

Another example is Medicare, which largely excludes preventive health services from its benefits. Prevention is now viewed as a major method for reducing morbidity at all ages, including old age. However, introducing benefits for prevention could result in increased costs, and the questions that need to be answered are the following: What are the health benefits that can be achieved through preventive measures? What are the effects on costs in introducing such benefits among the elderly?

The issue was considered of such importance that a study was mandated by Congress (Consolidated Omnibus Budget Reconciliation Act, 1985). The decision to use RCTs to answer the question was dictated by the uncertainty that an effect could be shown among the elderly. Further, with the rising costs of health care, some were asking whether introduction of preventive services might indeed be too costly. Accordingly, the hypothesis is directed at both health benefits and costs of the care received by the elderly.

Ethics of an RCT

By now there are established principles that affect the ethics of epidemiologic studies and, in particular, RCTs (Coughlin and Beauchamp, 1996). Their development has involved international and national professional organizations, universities, and funding agencies, and the process of making judgments about the need to reword or revise the principles is ongoing. The important components that appear to be firm are not reviewed here, but anyone who engages in epidemiologic research should be familiar with them. One element in the ethics of an RCT that is taken up in this chapter is whether the study group will experience a risk that would result in harm. This issue is of prime importance to the candidates for the planned experiment, but an answer is also needed for the physician and administrator, who make the decision of whether the experiment should move ahead. In the intervention involving low birth weight infants, the question is whether bringing these children in for day care at 12 months of age is hazardous because of the danger of exposure to communicable disease in such settings. Special measures were taken to reduce the risk to infants and parents, and the provider could be reassured on this score.

In the case of the Medicare preventive services trial, there is virtually no risk involved. However, there are many RCTs where the possibility of significant risk exists, and a strong case needs to be made about potential benefits. This held, for example, in testing the efficacy of lumpectomy for breast cancer, the decision to treat an experimental group of high-risk patients for breast cancer with tamoxifen, and the trial in the United Kingdom on whether certain patients with a myocardial infarction could be effectively treated at home instead of in the hospital. In both instances, the decision was to move ahead after considering the risks and benefits.

Not every question on intervention to improve the state of health of individuals can be subjected to an RCT. However, where an RCT is possible, we can ask whether it is indeed ethical not to conduct the RCT. A case in point concerns the large increase in the cesarean birth rate in the United States, from about 5% in the mid-1960s to 17% in 1980 and to 23% in the 1990s (National Center for Health Statistics, 1995). The necessity of a cesarean section in some of the births could have been debated and settled through an RCT. Instead, the field is dependent on data from observational studies that are far from definitive.

Functions of randomization: avoidance of bias and confounding

A major objective of randomization is to obtain two samples that have the same characteristics, thereby avoiding bias and confounding in the results. Bias at the time of entry into a trial occurs when the selection of the intervention and control groups lacks independence of exposure assignment from outcome assessment.

For example, in a study of clinic patients, should we decide to assign those who attend the morning sessions to the experimental group and those who attend the afternoon sessions to the control group or allocate those whose names are at the beginning of the alphabet to one group and the rest to the other group or assign patients of one set of primary care physicians to the experimental group and those under the care of another set of physicians to the control group?

Even though in each case care is taken to select at random an equal number from each subgroup, the experiment is not free of bias. Morning patients may be more acutely ill than those who appear in the afternoon; individuals whose names are at the beginning of the alphabet are more likely to belong to ethnic groups that differ from the others; the patients of one set of physicians may differ economically or socially from those of the other.

Bias also may occur through differential ascertainment of outcome in the intervention and control groups. This is readily apparent in studies of efficacy where outcome is based on survival rates and the opportunity to ascertain deaths is greater for one of the two groups. Another example of bias relates to the drop-out of individuals from the intervention group or the decision by some of the members of the control group to access the service being tested.

The problem of unequal ascertainment has no solution. If underascertainment is estimated as being larger for the intervention group than for the control group, a positive result in the trial can be judged as understating effectiveness. All other results leave the investigator uncertain of the experiment's results. Clearly, every effort must be made to avoid this type of bias.

Drop-outs and crossovers may be a more frequent source of bias. The issue is taken up below, but, by way of emphasis, it is necessary to point out that to maintain the integrity of the RCT, subjects are kept in the group to which they were randomized.

Confounding is most often thought of in connection with the analytic phase of a study, but it plays an important role in the rationale for structuring a study as an RCT.

Suppose we are interested in assessing the efficacy of an intervention aimed at the reduction of cholesterol for the control of myocardial infarctions. Age and degree of physical activity are possible confounding factors because both are associated with cholesterol level and the risk of myocardial infarction. In an RCT, it would be expected that the study and control groups would be balanced with respect to these confounding factors. Nevertheless, it would be important to check for this expectation. This step can be taken by comparing the experimental and control groups in their distributions of age and physical activity. If they are the same, then confounding by age and physical activity is not a source for concern; if they are not, it becomes necessary to handle this in the analysis.

Methods of randomization, comparability of study and control groups, and stratification

In an RCT, the experimental and control groups need to be drawn from the same frame of a defined universe or set of subjects. The unit of randomization is most often the individual, but it can be a geographic area, hospital, physician practice, or other type of cluster.

What are the methods through which this can be achieved?

This does not have a single answer. It can be accomplished through a simple random sample procedure (assignment based on the table of random numbers), a systematic random sample (assignment of the nth case to the study group and the $n + $ 1st case to the control group in a file not biased because of the order in which the cases have been entered), and assignment by the day of the month when the individual was born.

There are occasions when it is not feasible to start with a sampling of individuals, even though we are interested in an analysis of individuals. We may start with the selection of, for example, a random sample of hospitals or of geographic areas (referred to as "clusters") and then draw a sample of individuals within each of the selected clusters.

> *How can we assure ourselves that the intervention and control groups are equally balanced on certain characteristics?*

The approach taken is to stratify the universe from which the sample is to be drawn by characteristics that are known (or suspected) to be closely correlated with the outcome. These are usually labeled "prerandomization variables" (e.g., age, race/ethnicity, or sex). Sampling within strata increases the likelihood that the sample selected will be precisely the same in the study and control groups with respect to the characteristics stratified. However, there are many important variables in addition to the relatively few we may select for stratification. For these, we are dependent on randomization to achieve comparability.

To increase our confidence that comparability was actually achieved, samples of the intervention and control groups are often surveyed on a substantial number of characteristics to determine whether randomization, in fact, did work. If there is an intake or baseline interview, then the information can be obtained without the use of a special survey.

Volunteers vs. sampling from a defined population

Thus far, the discussion has been in terms of sampling from a population, starting with a listing of individuals or known clusters in which we have the opportunity to allocate subjects at random to an intervention or control group. However, frequently, this is not possible, and the sampling frame may have to consist of volunteers obtained through advertising, referrals by friends or physicians, etc.

> *Do we give anything up when we make the selection based on volunteers?*

In a study based on volunteers, we are effectively starting with a group that has agreed to be part of the experiment, and the allocation does not have to contend with the problem of refusals, a real advantage.

To avoid the possibility that volunteers will consist of a biased group with respect to such characteristics as age, sex, socioeconomic status, or health care behavior and attitudes, criteria that include some of these factors are established for admission to the trial. The problem that arises is that it is not feasible to extend the criteria to cover many of the variables. Attention then is directed to a more complete set of information obtained at the baseline of the trial. Conclusions from the RCT are limited to the extent that these data indicate that the sample departs from a general population.

> *In drawing a random sample from a defined population, to what extent do we really eliminate this problem?*

The issue comes down to the frequency of refusals. Refusal to participate may occur either at the point at which subjects are asked to enter the sampling frame or after their allocation to the intervention or control group. A judgment (or, if possible, a prior pilot study) is necessary to estimate the degree to which refusals will occur. If this is large and the study would be severely handicapped by refusals, the choice may have to be the use of a sample of volunteers. An expected modest proportion of refusers is reassuring, but for complete reassurance, it is best to check, to the degree possible, the characteristics of the acceptors with those of the refusers.

Contamination in an RCT (crossovers and drop-outs)

"Once randomized, always randomized." The most general interpretation of this aphorism is that, after randomization, each subject remains in the study or control group assigned at the beginning of the experiment.

> *What are the dangers in overlooking this principle?*

Common experiences include failure to continue to participate in the intervention because the individual changes his or her mind or the condition requires a change in treatment (e.g., an inability to tolerate the medication in a chemotherapeutic trial). Compelling as the reason may appear, either dropping the patient from the study or shifting the assignment to the control group would cause biases and jeopardize the results. In many studies, some observations can be derived for these drop-outs or crossovers, but they remain in the group to which they were assigned at the time of randomization.

The counterpart to this situation concerns crossovers by members of the control group who obtain services comparable to the intervention. This may occur in screening trials where some of the controls seek out the screening test if it is available in the general community.

Increasingly, it is recognized that the extent to which crossovers and drop-outs are likely to occur should be taken into account in determining the sample size. Actually, the issue can be of sufficient importance to call for a pilot study, on the basis of which judgments are made about the likely magnitude of nonparticipation by the study group and crossover by the control group.

Size of sample

After a decision is made to conduct an RCT, we are faced with the following question: Does the intervention have an effect large enough to make a difference in policy or planning? The answer to this question often dictates the size of the experiment, and the issue is faced prior to the start of the RCT.

Three types of information are required: the expected experience in the control group, the change that the experiment is designed to achieve, and the magnitude of two types of error we wish to avoid. Type 1 error (alpha) "consists of declaring that the difference in proportions (or rates) being studied is real when in fact the difference does not meet a standard generally agreed as statistically significant." Type 2 error (beta) "consists of failing to declare the two proportions (or rates) significantly different when in fact they are different" (Fleiss, 1981, pp. 32–34).

Alpha is often set at $p = 0.05$, and, most frequently, the model calls for a two-tailed test; a single-tailed test can be justified if it is known that the effect of the intervention cannot be negative. The power of the sample $(1 - \text{beta})$ tells us the chance of correctly concluding that the two proportions differ. In other words, it represents the probability that we will not miss detecting the difference being tested simply because of the size of the sample. The power of the sample is usually set at 0.80–0.90.

A number of computer software packages are available for estimation. Also, many textbooks on statistical methods contain tables that provide sample sizes for the intervention and control groups under varying conditions: a two-tailed test on proportions that differ in magnitude, alpha values of different size, and varying levels of power. For discussions of the derivation of sample size at specified levels of alpha, the power of the sample, and the other parameters of the problem, see Fleiss (1981) and Kraemer and Thiemann (1987).

Duration of an RCT

Frequently, the hypothesis of the RCT specifies the duration of the trial. For example, the efficacy of the interventions in the RCT involving low birth weight infants was to be judged when the children reached 3 years of age. However, the situation is different when we seek to establish an effect but no time limit is set. What are the strategies that can be used?

A particularly useful guide in this case is to designate the number of events the control group must accumulate before a firm conclusion is reached about the efficacy of the trial. This should be closely related to the expected number of events in the control group used in deriving the sample size. However, since we often operate on the basis of assumptions and these may be wrong, we may need to recalculate the duration of the trial using the actual experience of the control group to guide us.

Frequently, long-term follow-up is ruled out for administrative reasons. This is the situation in the trial to determine the efficacy of Medicare's waiving the costs for preventive health services among its beneficiaries. It is an open question whether a rapid change in the health condition of the intervention group relative to the control group can be expected in a short interval of time. However, a suggestion of the direction of change might be expected, and the results would need to be viewed as exploratory.

Interpretation of results

The value of an RCT for public policy and planning purposes is directly related to the generalizability of the results. Most often the intervention is tested in a single study, meaning that a single population group with perhaps special characteristics is observed. This is particularly true when the study is dependent on volunteers. Experience has shown that the most effective way to deal with this problem is through replication of the intervention trial or the organization of multiple trials conducted simultaneously.

One hopes and, in fact, expects that the results of the RCT will be relevant for a long time. However, external conditions during a trial can affect significantly the results.

Suppose a trial to determine the efficacy of a managed care program aimed at changing utilization practices is made available to a random sample of people in an underserved area. During the conduct of the study a new clinic is opened in the area. The net result could be to have the control group affected more by this change than the study group. Accordingly, we must pay attention not only to how the intervention is being administered but also to changes that occur in the environment of the study that may affect the actions of the individuals. It would be most unusual for the changes to be so large that the experiment had to be abandoned, but the results would have to be described in terms of what had occurred and, if possible, through a supplemental inquiry into the magnitude of the effect of the change.

Multiple interventions and multiple outcomes

In health services research, very often, it is necessary to determine simultaneously the efficacy or effectiveness of a set of interventions.

Can we assess the contribution of each of the interventions to the outcome?

This is an interesting question because of the challenge it poses for the interpretation of the results. We may want to assess the data in terms of the strength of each component of the intervention in producing an effect. However, the investigators, having committed the trial to an intervention that consists of multiple components, must contend with the fact that the interventions may be interacting or reinforcing each other in unspecified ways. This does not mean that we blind ourselves to the success or failure of implementing the interventions, and a critically important aspect of a trial is knowledge of the extent to which the interventions were delivered.

It may turn out that participation in one or more of the interventions was negligible, and it would seem reasonable to conclude that the remaining intervention(s) was responsible for the effect. The more usual situation is for all aspects of the interventions to be activated, though there may be diversity in the proportion of subjects who participate in one or another of the interventions. In this case, we have a less ambiguous situation, and the results of the trial are attributed to the combined set of interventions.

Two Case Examples

Two papers on two RCTs are summarized below for critical examination, utilizing the issues that arise when an RCT is being planned and during its conduct. Initial publications on the trials are covered, and methodology is given particular attention. At key points, questions are raised about the RCT's adherence or departure from the principles taken up. Also, at the end of each discussion, a series of questions is raised that should be answerable from the preceding material.

The senior health watch demonstration

Background. In 1985, Congress included in the Consolidated Omnibus Budget Reconciliation Act (COBRA) a section entitled "Demonstration of Preventive Health Services under Medicare" (COBRA, 1985). This instructed the Health Care Financing Administration (HCFA) to establish a 4-year "demonstration program designed to reduce disability and dependency through the provision of preventive health services" among Medicare beneficiaries. Medicare was oriented to the care of illness, and there were very few benefits of a preventive nature (pneumococcal pneumonia and hepatitis B immunizations).

The HCFA selected five sites nationally to evaluate the effectiveness and cost of comprehensive coverage of preventive and health risk screening services provided at no cost to the patient twice at annual intervals. Each site had the responsibility of designing and evaluating its intervention study; a central evaluation, covering all five sites, was to be conducted by an independent group. The experience in one of the sites, located in the eastern district of Baltimore, is discussed here. It was the only urban site that selected a broad base of community residents, with covered preventive services from the individuals' primary care providers.

Hypotheses and study design. The demonstration project was designed as a randomized controlled study. It was hypothesized that the offer of preventive services would be sufficiently attractive to the Medicare beneficiaries to elicit a large response rate; favorable effects on health would begin to become evident by the end of a follow-up period of 2 years, but savings due to the intervention would not appear during the 2-year interval because of the anticipated detection and treatment of previously unknown conditions. The project was later extended to include a second evaluation scheduled at the end of 4 years. The control group received the booklet *Strategies for Good Health,* published by the American Association of Retired Persons (AARP), which discusses prevention and offers guidance for those wishing further help in securing preventive services.

The preventive services package was based primarily on recommendations of the U.S. Preventive Services Task Force (1989) for persons aged 65 years and older. Covered services included a physical examination, with history and evaluation; laboratory procedures and immunizations; and counseling for health risks. Physicians were asked to review health risks; provide counseling where appropriate; take a complete history, including vision, hearing, and dentition; and include in the physical examination, breast, pelvic, and digital rectal examinations. Laboratory examinations included in the visit were total cholesterol, occult blood in stool, and a cervical smear (Papanicolaou test).

A fixed payment of $145 was provided for the clinic visit and laboratory tests; if a special follow-up counseling service was provided within 6 months of the clinic visit, the physician was reimbursed an additional $40. An encounter form was submitted by the physician, indicating procedures performed, health behaviors discussed, laboratory tests ordered, new problems, referrals for specialty care, and whether an additional counseling session was recommended.

Medicare services and allowable charges were obtained from Part A claims (acute hospital, skilled nursing facilities, home health, and hospice) and Part B claims (primarily charges for physician services in office and hospital settings). Additional patient information on sociodemographic characteristics, use of health services, and health status using the Quality of Well Being (QWB) scale and the General Health Questionnaire (GHQ) was obtained by telephone interview at the time of enrollment and later.

The QWB scale includes the assessment of symptoms, mobility, and physical and social activity; the score ranges from 0 to 1 (Kaplan and Anderson, 1988). The GHQ measures current emotional distress and the probability of an underlying mental disorder. The version used was the 28-item scale; a score of 0–4 was categorized as "no problem," 5–9 as a moderate problem, and 10 or greater as a severe problem (Goldberg and Hillier, 1978). Change in health was defined primarily as the difference in score of the QWB scale from enrollment to the 2-year interview. Four years after enrollment, a final telephone interview was held, covering the same items of information (results not available at this writing).

The potential benefits of the program were judged to exceed by far the risks faced by the subjects. The intervention group was assured that refusal would be at no penalty to them. Participants understood that selection for the preventive services was to be random.

Volunteers vs. sampling from a defined universe. The objectives of the study were to determine the responsiveness of the elderly population to participate in a prevention trial and to assess the effectiveness and costs of the intervention offered. This meant that sampling had to be based on a defined subgroup of Medicare beneficiaries living in a particular area. To call for volunteers would have negated the possibility of measuring the rate of participation in the trial.

The trial began with screening of the sample for eligibility, followed by a baseline survey, after which study subjects were randomly assigned to control or intervention groups. The overall completion rate in the telephone interviews with beneficiaries who were eligible for the project was 84%; 2,105 persons were designated as intervention cases and 2,090 persons as controls.

Contamination. The extent to which the intervention group activated its preventive health service benefit is discussed below under "Results and interpretation." Some in the control group may have had a similar type of service, but it was not expected that this would be a large number because of the additional payment this would have required. In any event, comparisons involving effectiveness, utilization of services, and costs are in terms of total intervention and total control groups.

Power of sample and duration of experiment. Power calculations were carried out under the assumption that the sample should have a power of 0.80 to detect a differential of ± 0.05, in a proportion of 0.50, using a two-tailed Type 1 error of 0.05. The number required in each of the intervention and control groups was 1,605. Allowance was made for failure to complete interviews and for attrition due to mortality after the study started.

Soon after the start of the study, provision was made for a final assessment through telephone interviews 4 years after randomization, though no extension was made for additional clinic visits or counseling services.

Results and interpretation. About 63% of the intervention group made a preventive clinical visit following the baseline interviews (German et al., 1995). About half of them returned for follow-up counseling within 6 months. There was a drop-off in the second preventive visit and the counseling visit that followed.

Participation in preventive visits varied only modestly, by characteristic of subject, but the direction of the variation was, on the main, as expected: participation decreased among those at the most advanced ages; it increased among the married, those who had a confidant, males, and those who had more than a grade school education; and contrary to most utilization literature, nonwhites were more likely to go for such visits than whites. Past preventive care and current health behaviors made a difference in participation. Of those with middle QWB scores, 66% went for visits compared with 57% of those with low scores and 58% of those with high scores. Accordingly, both the sickest and the healthiest individuals were less likely to go for preventive services.

Patients with providers in solo practice and those with female providers were more likely to make a preventive visit. Very few patients reported hospital-based physicians as their source of primary care. Logistic regressions showed, among males, higher odds ratios for making visits for those who were married and had clinicians in private practice (Table 9-1). Among females, having a confidant,

Table 9-1. Odds ratios for characteristics associated with preventive visits in a logistic regression model, Senior Health Watch Demonstration

	Odds Ratio	95% Confidence Interval
Men		
Married	1.52	1.09–2.08
Type of practice of provider[a]		
Solo	1.95	1.38–2.75
Hospital	4.35	0.92–20.52
Women		
Having a confidant	1.53	1.13–2.07
Having a female provider	1.93	1.21–3.08
Education[b]		
High school	1.34	1.04–1.71
College	1.33	0.91–1.97
Mammography[c]	1.75	1.38–2.23

[a]Comparison group was providers in group practices.

[b]Comparison group had 0–8 years of education.

[c]Reported having mammography within 2 years of baseline.

having a high school education, and having had a mammogram in the 2 years prior to baseline were positively associated with making a visit.

The intervention and control groups had similar QWB scores at baseline (0.712 and 0.709, respectively), and there were no between-group differences in other indicators of health, including number of disability days, number of hospital days in the past year, and self-evaluation of health. Mean change scores over the 2-year period showed that the intervention group declined less, 0.06 points compared with 0.08 points for controls ($p = 0.01$). This difference is primarily a result of a higher proportion of deaths in the control group (231/2,090, 11.1/100, controls; 175/2,105, 8.3/100, intervention group). Linear regression analysis showed that those in the group offered intervention were in better health at 2 years, controlling for other variables affecting health. There was an interaction between education and intervention: persons with lower education benefitted more than those with higher education.

Utilization and costs. Contrary to expectation, the total allowable Medicare charges were somewhat higher for the control group in the first year, even when payments for preventive services were included for the intervention (Table 9-2) (Burton et al., 1995). In the second year, allowable charges plus other costs were 2.5% higher for the control group than the intervention group. The savings expected for the intervention group over the longer term appear to be occurring in the second year.

Hospital discharge rates per 1,000 were lower for the intervention group in the 2 years (Table 9-3). However, controls had shorter hospital stays. Patients in the intervention group had somewhat lower rates of office visits, but a slightly higher proportion in the intervention group made an ambulatory visit than in the control group.

Conclusions and questions. In a representative group of Medicare eligibles in the type of community studied, approximately two-thirds would take advantage over a 2-year period of the opportunity to be seen by their primary care physician for a preventive visit. A slight improvement in health status would occur, and the result would be little or no impact on charges under Medicare for all offered the visits.

The level of participation is judged to be a positive finding given the fact that a random sample of Medicare beneficiaries at all ages, regardless of their health status, was studied. All were living in the community at the start of the demonstration project and not in nursing homes or other institutions. The effects of preventive services on general health were small and due to the lower death rate in the intervention group. Several explanations for the lower death rate were

Table 9-2. Total charges by study group and by year, Senior Health Watch Demonstration

| | Medicare Part A | | Medicare | | | |
	Hospital Charges in Dollars	Other Charges in Dollars	Part B Charges in Dollars[a]	Cost of Intervention in Dollars[b]	Cost of Other Waivers in Dollars[c]	Total Dollars
			Year 1			
Intervention ($n = 2,105$)	5,027,343	366,571	3,239,659	190,865	1,640	8,826,078
Control ($n = 2,090$)	5,212,370	375,698	3,398,852		4,143	8,991,063
			Year 2			
Intervention ($n = 2,020$)	6,284,111	493,211	3,833,013	119,051	5,756	10,735,142
Control ($n = 1,971$)	6,355,516	674,761	3,976,499		7,423	11,014,199

[a] Part B claims are primarily physician claims for services in the office, hospital, nursing home, home, etc. Supplier and some laboratory charges are included in this type of claim.

[b] Preventive visits were reimbursed $145 and counseling visits $40.

[c] Charges for Medicare-covered services received by patients through a waivered program funded by the Health Care Financing Administration.

Table 9-3. Comparison of selected measures of utilization by study group and by study year, Senior Health Watch Demonstration

	Number	Discharges/1,000[a]	Mean Length of Stay (Days)	Mean Ambulatory Visits/Year[b]
		Year 1		
Intervention	2,105	345.6	12.4	6.5
Control	2,090	355.2	10.5	7.0
		Year 2		
Intervention	2,020	378.0	10.1	7.2
Control	1,971	404.4	9.9	7.2

[a] Adjusted from number of persons available for admission (enrolled and living) each month.

[b] Mean ambulatory visits per year were calculated as the number of visits each month directed by the number of persons enrolled and living that month multiplied by 12.

examined, with the final judgment being that none pointed toward an artifactual basis for this observation.

Findings with respect to costs and utilization were unexpected and positive. Usually, one expects to find an incremental cost associated with the provision of preventive services, but this did not occur. Whether or not there is a longer-term impact upon charges and utilization of services, as well as health status, will be examined on the basis of the follow-up interview at 4 years from randomization.

The demonstration project made available two prevention and two counseling visits 1 year apart; initially, the plan was to assess the impact of these services at the end of 2 years, later extended to 4 years. What was the underlying purpose of including a follow-up at the end of 4 years? Was this realistic since the intervention ended at the start of year 2?

In measuring the effect on utilization of ambulatory care, the visits made for prevention were included in the number of ambulatory care visits. An alternative might have been to exclude preventive health visits. What arguments do you see in favor of the approach taken? Would it have been advantageous to exclude the preventive visits?

About 63% of the intervention group made a preventive health visit, and all results were based on the total intervention group, including those who did not participate. Why was this done? Could the study have proceeded with measurements based on comparisons between the controls and the 63% of the intervention group? Why not?

What conclusions are justified on the basis of the 2 years of follow-up in this demonstration project? How important do you see the emphasis on showing outcome data by individual year from baseline? Why?

The health insurance experiment

Background. Concern about the access, costs, and quality of health care is not a new phenomenon. The issues involved in resolving the problems of inadequate access to care by some segments of the population, escalating costs for health services, and lags in health status of the population have occupied a dominant place on the political agenda of the country.

A question that has loomed large is whether coinsurance and deductibles in health insurance might not go a long way in dealing effectively with these issues. The proponents of coinsurance and deductibles have argued that they are needed to discourage overutilization and that this could be accomplished without significant effect on health status, while their opponents have generally feared that they may prevent necessary services from being obtained.

Early in the 1970s it was decided that the effect of different levels of cost sharing in health insurance on utilization, expenditures, and health status should be investigated and that this should be carried out through an RCT. Available were the findings of an observational study of the experience of subscribers to the Group Health Plan offered to Stanford University employees and their dependents, whose benefits had changed from no charge for clinic services in and out of the hospital and for extended hospital stays to a 25% coinsurance charge for clinic services (Scitovsky and Snyder, 1972; Scitovsky and McCall, 1977). The results suggested a decrease in utilization and costs.

Hypotheses and study design. The RCT was designed and carried out by the Health Sciences Program, The Rand Corporation, 1974–1982 (Newhouse, 1974). A dominant question was the extent to which health care services increase as cost sharing decreases. On both a theoretic and an empiric basis, it was expected that lower cost sharing would result in greater utilization. What needed particular inquiry was the gradient of this relation under different degrees of cost sharing, the sectors of health care (hospital or ambulatory care) most affected, and the extent to which socioeconomic characteristics of individuals influenced the results. Closely allied to these issues was whether having health insurance that covers all costs of health care leads to a healthier life than is the case for having insurance that requires cost sharing and whether prepaid group practice showed a special advantage.

Six sites were selected to represent the four census geographic regions of the country, with attention given to obtaining a spectrum of city sizes that would reflect the variation in delivery of health services and the demand for care. About 7,700 persons (2,756 families) were enrolled, 70% for 3 years, the rest for 5 years. The age group was 61 years or younger, thereby excluding persons who were already or would become eligible for Medicare before the end of the observation period; also excluded were individuals who were eligible for disability payments through Medicare and families with high incomes.

Four coinsurance plans were compared: 0% (free care), 25%, 50%, and 95% as the fraction of the bill paid by the family. The maximum dollar expenditure varied with family income, but there was a $1,000 maximum annually. One plan differed from the others: it had a 95% coinsurance rate, but the annual out-of-pocket expenditure was limited to $150 per person and $450 per family, which was viewed as approximating a plan with a $150 per person deductible (referred to as the "individual deductible plan"); cost sharing applied only to outpatient services, and inpatient services were free to the family. Dollar figures refer to conditions under which the experiment was carried out; no adjustments were made to update these figures.

Utilization and expenditure data were obtained from claims records (except in the case of the prepaid group practice, where medical records were reviewed for services received); personal characteristics were elicited through interviews; general health (such as physical health, role functioning, and health perceptions) and health habits (such as smoking) were collected from a self-administered questionnaire at enrollment and at the end of the study (3 or 5 years later); blood pressure, serum cholesterol level, and visual acuity were measured for a random sample of the enrollees at the start and end of the experiment.

Ethics of the program. Consent was obtained for participation in this experimental program. No changes were required from the participants in how they were to receive health services (except for those allocated to the prepaid group practice program); the only changes were in the copayment system to which they were allocated, and, in this case, they were not liable to lose financially compared with the health insurance plan to which they had belonged (enrollment in their prior plan was ensured at the end of the experiment).

Randomization. Of the contacted families in a community, 15% refused a screening or baseline interview; it is not known whether these families would have behaved differently from those who enrolled. Twenty percent of the families interviewed refused to participate. Their characteristics and prior use of medical care did not differ importantly from those who enrolled, and it was concluded that there was no bias in the results. To ensure comparability between the arms of the study, the distribution of 20 characteristics of families or individuals was made as similar as possible across insurance plans.

Volunteers vs. sampling from a defined universe. The multisite character of the experiment was designed to broaden the generalizability of the results, and the samples selected are representative of the communities where the families lived. Selection on the basis of volunteers would have raised questions about the reasons for volunteering and would have made it more difficult to draw conclusions from the experiment.

Contamination. Analysis included persons who participated in the experiment for the entire year being studied, including those who died during the year. About 95% of the persons initially enrolled in the experiment were retained in the sample; attrition was estimated to be 2–3% per year.

Power of sample. A multisite study was carried out in which several different types of health insurance plan were tested, without regard to power calculations. Similarity of results among the sites would increase the confidence of the results.

Results and interpretation. Total expenditure per capita rose steadily as coinsurance decreased (Newhouse et al., 1981a,b). The difference in expenditure per person was greatest between those with free coverage and those who had the 95% coinsurance plan (Table 9-4). Expenditure in the other plans fell between these two extremes. With few exceptions, in each site and year, expenditures for ambulatory services per person rose as coinsurance fell. Applying techniques that yielded predictions of what the expenditures would have been if a larger number of families had been enrolled indicated that the predicted expenditure in the 95% coinsurance plan was 69% of that in the free plan (i.e., free care results in 50% higher expenditure than 95% coinsurance).

Table 9-4. Actual annual total and ambulatory expenditure per person by plan in nine site-years,[a] Health Insurance Experiment

Plan	Total Expenditure in Dollars	Ambulatory Expenditure in Dollars
Free care	401 ± 52	186 ± 9
25% Coinsurance	346 ± 58	149 ± 10
50% Coinsurance	328 ± 149	120 ± 12
95% Coinsurance	354 ± 37	114 ± 10
Individual deductible, 95% coinsurance[b]	333 ± 74	140 ± 11

[a]Ninety-five percent confidence intervals are presented with expenditure data. Amounts are in current dollars, beginning in late 1974 and extending through late 1978. Numbers are uncorrected for price-level differences by site or for small differences in allocation to plan by site. The F value to test the null hypothesis of no differences among the plans in total expenditure is 3.14 ($p < 0.05$). The F value to test the null hypothesis of no differences among the plans in ambulatory expenditure is 33.4 ($p < 0.01$).

[b]Coinsurance in this plan applies to outpatient care only; inpatient care is free.

Full coverage led to more people using services and to more services per user. Both ambulatory services and hospital admissions increased (Table 9-5). However, once patients were admitted to the hospital, expenditures per admission did not differ significantly among the experimental plans.

Expenditure by adults showed greater responsiveness to variation in cost sharing than did expenditure for children. This occurred largely because hospitalization of children showed no significant response to plan, whereas hospitalization among adults was significantly higher in the free-care plan. In most of the sites participating in the experiment, different income groups had relatively similar responses.

The investigators interpret the results involving the individual deductible plan as tending to refute the argument that cost sharing, especially for ambulatory services, raises overall costs; this would occur by inducing persons to delay seeking care and encouraging physicians to hospitalize patients who could be treated on an outpatient basis. Another point made is that making care free does not appear to eliminate variation of use with income in most of the sites studied. The argument that full coverage may improve health, or that cost sharing induces persons to forego necessary services is counterpoised by the argument that the elimination of cost sharing will induce persons to consume unnecessary services or to seek care for trivial problems. This issue requires evidence on comparisons of health outcomes, that is taken up next.

The outcome phase of the study was restricted to persons aged 14–61 years at the start, 3,958 individuals (Brook et al., 1983). The principal question was whether the free plan improved health more than the cost-sharing plans. Of special interest was the effect of cost sharing on people with poor health or low income. For the average person in the experiment, the only significant effect of

Table 9-5. Annual probability of one or more visits to physicians or hospital admissions in nine site-years,[a] Health Insurance Experiment

Plan	Visits to Physicians	Hospital Admissions
Free care	0.84 ± 0.02	0.102 ± 0.013
25% Coinsurance	0.78 ± 0.03[b]	0.081 ± 0.014[c]
50% Coinsurance	0.75 ± 0.05[b]	0.072 ± 0.021[b]
95% Coinsurance	0.69 ± 0.04[b]	0.076 ± 0.014[b]
Individual deductible, 95% coinsurance[d]	0.73 ± 0.04[b]	0.090 ± 0.016

[a]Ninety-five percent confidence intervals are presented for all plans. Standard errors are corrected for intrafamily and intertemporal correlations.

[b]$p < 0.01$ compared with the free plan by the one-tailed test.

[c]$p < 0.05$.

[d]This plan has zero coinsurance (free care) for inpatient services.

free care ($p < 0.05$) was that for corrected far vision, though the difference in diastolic blood pressure approached statistical significance. However, in the free-care plan, the relative risk for dying (based on smoking habits, cholesterol level, and systolic blood pressure) was lower than for those in the cost-sharing plan. Improvements in vision, blood pressure, and risk of dying were largest in the group with low income and elevated risk (Table 9-6). No conclusion could be reached about the effect of free care on individuals with higher income and high risk.

The investigators reached three conclusions about the influence of free care on health status: (1) free care had no effect on the major health habits associated with cardiovascular disease and some types of cancer; (2) free care had no effect on the self-assessed measures of health used in the study (small samples made the conclusions regarding subgroups classified by income or initial state of health uncertain); and (3) people with specific conditions, which physicians have been trained to diagnose and treat, benefit from free care. In summary, they point out that poor families were protected by an income-related ceiling on their out-of-pocket medical expenditures.

Two additional questions were investigated in the Health Insurance Experiment:

> *When persons previously receiving care from fee-for-service physicians are randomly assigned to receive care at a prepaid group practice, how does their use differ from that of persons enrolled in fee-for-service insurance plans? How does the use of the former group differ from the use of persons already enrolled in the group practice plan?* (Manning et al., 1984).

The prepaid group practice studied, Group Health Cooperative of Puget Sound (GHC), in Seattle, was a well-established program of its type (a capitation pay-

Table 9-6. Differences between free and cost-sharing plans in predicted exit values of blood pressure and vision and the risk of dying, according to initial health status income, Health Insurance Experiment

| | Elevated Risk[a] | |
Physiologic Measures	Low Income	High Income
Diastolic blood pressure	-3.3 (-5.9 to -0.7)[b]	-0.4 (-2.6 to 1.8)
Functional far vision	-0.3 (-0.6 to 0.02)	-0.1 (0.4 to 0.2)
Risk of dying	-0.30 (-0.60 to -0.04)	-0.13 (-0.40 to 0.10)

[a]The mean value of diastolic blood pressure for persons at elevated risk is 88. For functional far vision, elevated risk refers only to the upper one-quarter of the distribution of values for uncorrected natural vision. The risk of dying from any cause is relative to that of persons with average values of major risk factors (smoking, cholesterol, systolic blood pressure). Predictions in these two columns were made with the mean value of the elevated risk group.

[b]Numbers in parentheses, 95% confidence intervals. All intervals that do not include 0 are significant at $p < 0.05$.

ment system with most services free of charge). Three groups were selected at random from the community for assignment: GHC (1,149 persons), free service (431 persons), and cost-sharing fee-for-service (782 persons). A fourth group consisted of a random sample of GHC individuals who had already been enrolled in the plan for at least 1 year (733 persons). In the case of utilization, GHC records were reviewed, and claims forms served as the source of information for the fee-for-service plans. In the case of physician services, comparisons were made using the California Relative Value Studies for the GHC and fee-for-service care delivered.

The experimental and control groups in GHC differed little in imputed expenditure on medical services, but they both differed markedly from the fee-for-service group (about 28% lower for the experimental group and 23% lower for the control group). Differences between the experience in GHC and in the free service group were due mainly to the lesser frequency of those in GHC being admitted to the hospital. There were 40% fewer admissions in the two GHC samples than in the free services plan. All cost-sharing plans had both lower admission rates and lower visit rates than the free service plan.

A principal conclusion was that, because of the experimental design of the study, the observation of much less hospitalization among participants at GHC than among those in the free service plan adds weight to findings in observational studies. The experimental group and the control group in GHC had very similar experiences. This lays to rest, at least for this program, the speculation that the plan's lower hospital rates may be due to selection of more favorable groups at the time of enrollment.

The investigators observed increases in the GHC sample only in bed-days and serious symptoms, and these differences were confined to the low-income, initially sick group (not shown) (Ware et al., 1986). Those in the top 40% of the income distribution who began the experiment with health problems had significantly lower cholesterol levels and significantly better general health ratings in GHC than in the free service. Thus, for the economically advantaged, there were two reasons to encourage enrollment in the health maintenance organization (HMO) studied: substantial cost savings and gains in health status. The low-income group who began the experiment with health problems appeared worse off at GHC by comparison with free and fee-for-service groups.

In commenting on the significance of the favorable findings for low-income participants in the fee-for-service plans, the investigators speculate that this may not hold for the poor on Medicaid. Because many physicians did not accept Medicaid patients, due to lower reimbursement, health outcomes in both the free and fee-for-service groups might be better than those for the poor in the Medicaid program area. Nevertheless, the investigators caution that, with many states considering mandatory prepaid arrangements to reduce or contain Medicaid expenditures, special provisions may be needed to minimize the possibility that HMOs achieve cost savings for the poor with health problems at the expense of health.

> *Many changes have taken place since the 1970s when the experiment took place, for example, increase in cost of health care that exceeded cost of living in general, growth of HMOs, decreases in hospital admissions rates at all ages, etc. What limitations do these impose on the interpretation of the results?*

> *The first paper on the study's results was on the topic of utilization and costs. A major question raised in an editorial was whether the higher figures for the free care group vs. the coinsurance groups reflected too much health care (among those with free care) or too little (among those with coinsurance). Can the question be answered with the results that came out later on health status? In what way? What problems do you see dealing with this issue?*

> *A significant component of the trial was the inclusion of a comparison between GHC, an HMO, and fee-for-service health insurance. How far can we go in generalizing the observations from this study?*

> *In the Health Insurance Experiment, subjects were allocated at random to different experimental groups; in real life, families select the type of health insurance coverage they prefer from among the plans available to them. What messages does this experiment have for the families making the choices?*

Conclusions

The two examples of the application of the RCT illustrate the strengths of this methodology and the compromises that are often necessary. Randomization added confidence that the comparisons were between highly comparable groups except for the intervention and that the problems of bias and confounding could be dismissed as irrelevant in assessing the results.

A significant handicap in RCTs is the time limitation often set for the intervention. Both of the examples were under this constraint. In the National Insurance Experiment, it may have been desirable to extend the study beyond the time limit set, but the duration was long enough to draw useful conclusions. In the Medicare study, it was known at the start that the time frame for the intervention might be too brief. In this sense then, the study was at risk, and the question is whether the risk should have been accepted. In the phase of the study conducted in Baltimore, some answers could be obtained about the early impact of the interventions on health status and costs, but the results leave important issues unanswered.

Generalizability is enhanced when it becomes possible to conduct a trial on a multisite basis. To a large extent, the results of the National Insurance Experiment overcame one of the major criticisms of RCTs: the fact that they are often single-sited and, therefore, may be limited by special circumstances or population characteristics. This is the restriction in the interpretation of the National Insurance Experiment's application of an RCT to determine differences in outcome between enrollment in an HMO (prepaid group practice) and coverage by fee-for-service insurance. However, this limitation does not obviate the value of the results for the HMO component of the study, which reconfirmed reductions in hospital costs in HMOs and gave support to the proposition that such a favorable finding was not due to selection bias in enrollment of individuals.

Although several sites were involved in the Medicare study, each had a different methodology, and, while it is possible to obtain an overview of the impact of the availability of preventive services for the older population, major differences do exist and caution is needed in the interpretation of the consolidated results. The Baltimore study represents an application to a single site and is of interest because of the methodology in which a random sample of a community of Medicare beneficiaries was included.

References

Brook, R. H., J. E. Ware, W. H. Rogers, et al. 1983. Does free care improve adults' health? Results from a randomized controlled trial. *N. Engl. J. Med.,* 309:1426–1434.

Burton, L. C., D. M. Steinwachs, P. S. German, et al. 1995. Preventive services for the elderly: would coverage affect utilization and costs under Medicare? *Am. J. Public Health,* 85:387–391.

Consolidated Omnibus Budget Reconciliation Act of 1985 (COBRA). Public law 99-272, sec. 9314.

Coughlin, S. S., and T. L. Beauchamp. 1996. *Ethics and Epidemiology.* New York: Oxford University Press.

Fisher, B., and C. Redmond. 1992. Lumpectomy for breast cancer: an update of the NSABP experience. National Surgical Adjuvant Breast and Bowel Project. *Monogr. Natl. Cancer Inst.,* 11:7–13.

Fleiss, J. L. 1981. Determining sample sizes needed to detect a difference between two proportions. In: *Statistical Methods for Rates and Proportions,* 2nd ed. New York: John Wiley & Sons, pp. 33–49.

Freis, E. D. 1967. Effects of treatment on morbidity in hypertension. Results in patients with diastolic blood pressures averaging 115 through 129 mm Hg. *JAMA,* 202:116–122.

German, P. S., L. Burton, S. Shapiro, et al. 1995. Extended coverage for preventive services for the elderly: response and results in a demonstration population. *Am. J. Public Health,* 85:379–386.

Goldberg, D. P., and V. F. Hillier. 1978. A scaled version of the general health questionnaire. *Psychol. Med.,* 9:139–145.

Kaplan, R. M., and J. P. Anderson. 1988. A general health policy model; update and applications. *Health Serv. Res.,* 23:203–235.

Kemper, P. 1988. Overview of the findings. The evaluation of the National Long Term Care Demonstration, 10. *Health Serv. Res.,* 23:161–174.

Kraemer, H. C., and S. Thiemann. 1987. *How Many Subjects? Statistical Power Analysis in Research.* Newbury Park, CA: Sage Publications.

Last, J. M. 1988. *A Dictionary of Epidemiology,* 2nd ed., edited by J. M. Last. New York: Oxford University Press.

Manning, W. G., A. Leibowitz, G. A. Goldberg, et al. 1984. A controlled trial of the effect of a prepaid group practice on use of services. *N. Engl. J. Med.,* 310:1505–1510.

Multiple Risk Factor Intervention Trial Group. 1977. Statistical design considerations in the NHLI Multiple Risk Factor Intervention Trial (MRFIT). *J. Chron. Dis.,* 20:261–275.

A Multisite, Randomized Trial. 1990. Enhancing the outcomes of low-birth-weight, premature infants. The Infant Health and Development Program. *JAMA,* 263:3035–3042.

National Center for Health Statistics. 1995. *Health, United States, 1994.* Hyattsville, MD: U.S. Public Health Service, Table 88.

Newhouse, J. P. 1974. A design for a health insurance experiment. *Inquiry,* 11:5–27.

Newhouse, J. P., W. G. Manning, C. N. Morris, et al. 1981a. *Some Interim Results from a Controlled Trial of Cost Sharing in Health Insurance.* Santa Monica, CA: Rand Corporation.

Newhouse, J. P., W. G. Manning, C. N. Morris, et al. 1981b. Some interim results from a controlled trial of cost sharing in health insurance. *N. Engl. J. Med.,* 305:1501–1507.

Scitovsky, A. A., and N. McCall. 1977. Coinsurance and the demand for physician services: four years later. *Soc. Secur. Bull.,* 40:19–27.

Scitovsky, A. A., and N. M. Snyder. 1972. Effect of coinsurance on use of physician services. *Soc. Secur. Bull.,* 35:3–19.

Streptomycin in Tuberculosis Trials Committee. 1948. Streptomycin treatment of pulmonary tuberculosis. *Br. Med. J.,* 2:769–782.

U.S. Preventive Services Task Force. 1989. *Guide to Clinical Preventive Services: An Assessment of the Effectiveness of 169 Interventions.* Baltimore: Williams & Wilkins.

Ware, J. E., Jr., R. H. Brook, W. H. Rogers, et al. 1986. Comparison of health outcomes at a health maintenance organization with those of fee-for-service care. *Lancet,* 1:1017–1022.

CHAPTER 10

Screening for Secondary Prevention of Disease

SAM SHAPIRO

Prevention of disease and relief from distress due to adverse health conditions have been major objectives of public health. Primary prevention that seeks to eliminate specific diseases and other departures from good health is central to goals in the field of public health. Immunization against childhood diseases, antismoking campaigns, and reduction of environmental pollutants are examples of long-standing activities in which the practitioners of public health have exerted great influence.

The special roles of other forms of prevention have gained visibility. Secondary prevention that aims at early detection and prompt and effective interventions to correct departures from good health has been particularly relevant for the control of several types of cancer. Tertiary prevention that is directed at reducing or eliminating long-term impairments and disabilities and extends prevention into the field of rehabilitation has applications for many health conditions and special value as people advance in age.

Attention is focused in this chapter on screening and its relevance for secondary prevention of different types of cancer. Screening has the special function of sorting out apparently well persons who probably have a disease from those who do not. The test of screening's value for prevention is to establish its efficacy, i.e., whether its use leads to lowered mortality from the cancer being targeted. The positive and negative effects of screening on quality of life are important, but, in the end, saving lives has been the primary concern in cancer screening because of the high lethal consequences of the condition.

The early part of the chapter considers the following:

- major issues that affect our thinking about the value of screening
- guidelines for considering the state of readiness of introducing screening
- the importance of balancing benefits and risks, costs, and effectiveness in screening
- the strength of different methods in measuring the effectiveness of screening

183

As discussed in other chapters, epidemiology provides an array of research methods for studying the efficacy of an intervention. The complexity of decisions in adopting an intervention and the role of epidemiologic methods in those decisions are illustrated in this chapter. In the particular set of cancer sites to be taken up here, there is wide agreement that the randomized controlled trial (RCT) is the most relevant. However, it is unlikely that all of the issues that need settling will be resolved. Two cancers, breast and colorectal, reviewed in this chapter are based on RCTs that have been applied; their results are positive for screening, but questions remain.

It is expected that, with the aid of questions in each section of the chapter, the reader will recognize not only the rationale for the use of the RCT in testing the efficacy of screening but also the nature of the issues that have to be dealt with in moving from a trial to application in society.

Guiding Principles for the Development of Screening

An important impetus to research in the field of screening was the clarification of the requirements for its application in a population (Wilson and Jungren, 1968). These can be summarized as follows.

1. The condition screened for is an important cause of morbidity, disability, or mortality.
2. The natural history of the disease is sufficiently well known; risks from screening are low enough; and efficacy in reducing morbidity, disability, or mortality is high enough to conclude that (a) detection of the disease through screening will lead to a net benefit to the target population and (b) the resources required to administer the tests under screening conditions are justified in terms of the net benefits.
3. The tests must have high levels of sensitivity and specificity, where ''sensitivity'' is defined as the proportion with the disease who are positive to the test and ''specificity'' as the proportion without the disease who are negative to the test.
4. The tests must be acceptable to the target population and their health care providers, and appropriate follow-up of positive findings must be ensured.

What rules can we derive from these principles that would convince us to introduce population-wide screening?

In answering this question, we have to face the fact that there are no absolute standards to determine when these conditions have been met or how to combine them to reach a decision. All are stated in relative terms, and a specific disease may rate extremely high in significance in mortality but only moderately high on the basis of knowledge about its natural history. The point is that value judgments play a large role in weighing the relative importance of the above conditions. However, the most compelling of all principles in the decision of whether screening should be advocated for a population is the need to demonstrate efficacy of the procedure.

Benefits and Risks

Screening is expected to result in more frequent detection of cancer during a preinvasive stage or in an earlier stage of invasive disease than is usual in clinical practice. The immediate benefit is less extensive treatment, thereby reducing the discomfort and disability that impair physical and social functioning.

What problems are there in screening that we have to be aware of?

One concern is that, as screening procedures increase their capacity to detect cancer close to the onset of the disease, we may be detecting some cases that would otherwise never be manifested clinically. Furthermore, earlier detection through screening means earlier awareness that cancer is present and additional years of monitoring the condition and anxiety about the course of the disease, the psychologic and behavioral effects of which are largely unknown. To the extent that clear evidence exists that intervention decreases the likelihood of occurrence of invasive disease or the long-term risk of more advanced disease, and thereby its associated mortality, such concerns are reduced.

Choice of the RCT for Testing Efficacy

Large investments in RCTs have been justified as the most certain way to obtain a suitable comparison group to determine whether and by how much screening reduces mortality from the cancer being targeted. Other methodologies have been used, for example, case-control and longitudinal observational studies. However, these have been applied primarily in situations where it has not been possible to conduct an RCT or where special circumstances dictated their application.

What are some of the factors that have led to the conclusion that the RCT should be used whenever possible?

Although the natural history of the disease after clinical detection may be known, extrapolating from this knowledge to cases detected by screening, even after considering the stage of disease, is not as straightforward as it seems. In fact, the following question may be asked: Why not use comparisons of survival rates instead of comparisons of mortality rates, where "survival rates" represent the proportion of individuals with cancer who survive a defined time period and "mortality rates" the proportion of a population who die from cancer in a defined time period?

Two circumstances impose special difficulties in the interpretation of survival rates based on cases detected in the group invited for screening vs. cases detected through usual clinical practice. These are lead time and length-biased sampling, both defined below. They are subject to measurement error, but death rates avoid the problems they impose.

Lead time gained in detecting cancer by screening is the interval of time screening brings the detection of a case closer to the date of origin of the disease than would occur in clinical practice. Accordingly, case survival over x years in clinical practice is the equivalent to case survival over that amount of time (x) in years plus the lead time gained through screening (y) and length-biased sampling, that is, the propensity of screening to result in the detection of slower growing tumors. Length-biased sampling distinguishes between cases by their rate of growth, whereas lead time measures how much sooner a case is detected through screening. Faster growing tumors have less of a chance to be detected on screening and a poorer prognosis than slower growing cases. Case survival rates, therefore, would be biased in favor of the cases detected through screening.

Other conditions include the uncertainty about how the natural history of the disease varies by characteristics of the population and the possibility that volunteers for screening may have different underlying prognoses from the rest of the population. These factors make it imperative to have a suitable comparison group when studies are being designed, to determine the efficacy of a screening procedure. However, there will still be a question about how to extrapolate from a study of volunteers to the general population.

Precision

Balancing benefits against risks involves the sensitivity and specificity of the screening procedures. The fact that screening sorts out apparently well persons who probably have a disease from those who probably do not means that there will inevitably be false-positive and false-negative results. These arise from limitations in the screening technology, misinterpretation of screening results, and differences among physicians on the course of action to be taken.

How serious a problem is this? In the first place, false-positive results lead to unnecessary confirmatory additional diagnostic workup, which may vary from relatively minor to extensive procedures. These add to the cost and cause discomfort and increased anxiety. Second, false-negative results reduce the effectiveness of screening to achieve its primary goal of reduced mortality from cancer, threaten loss in confidence of the procedure among physicians and the population, and could cause patient delay in seeking care when symptoms do appear

Table 10-1. Measurement of sensitivity, specificity, and positive predictive value of screening for cancer

		Cancer Confirmation		
		+	−	Total
Screening Test	+	a	b	$a + b$
	−	c	d	$c + d$
	Total	$a + c$	$b + d$	

$$\text{Sensitivity} = \frac{a}{a + c}$$

$$\text{Specificity} = \frac{d}{b + d}$$

$$\text{Positive Predictive Value} = \frac{a}{a + b}$$

(i.e., unless the results of a negative examination are bolstered by information about the need to respond to symptoms between screening examinations).

Table 10-1 gives the derivation of sensitivity and specificity ratios; also included are the positive predictive values that are derivable from the experience in a screening program (negative predictive values are not shown for they are extremely high).

Table 10-2 shows the results of different levels of sensitivity and specificity on what we see in screening for cancer with an incidence rate of 5/1,000. In the upper half of this table, a relatively low specificity, 85%, is accepted to achieve a high sensitivity, 90%. Approximately 15% of the subjects are referred for additional examinations, and the positive predictive value of screening is low, 2.9%. The negative predictive value is high, close to 100%, as would be expected in this example, where the incidence rate is 5/1,000, even though the specificity rate is characterized as relatively low, 85%.

Table 10-2. Effect of varying sensitivity and specificity on referrals and predictive values of screening for cancer

High sensitivity, low specificity, incidence (5/1,000)	
Se = 90%	Sp = 85%
Referred = 15%	PPV = 2.9%
Low sensitivity, high specificity, incidence (5/1,000)	
Se = 65%	Sp = 98%
Referred = 2.3%	PPV = 14%

Se, sensitivity; Sp, specificity; PPV, positive predictive value.

In the lower half of the table, high specificity, 98% is sought at the expense of lowered sensitivity, 65%. This causes a reverse situation in which 2.3% are referred for additional examinations and the positive predictive value is 14%; the negative predictive value is again very high, almost 100%. The burden on the participants and the costs are affected heavily by the levels of these values. Finally, if choices can be made, a key consideration is the effect of these levels on screening acceptance by the population and physicians and on reductions in mortality achievable through screening.

A point to bear in mind is that a reduction in mortality in a screening program is dependent on the level of the sensitivity rate: a high rate will more clearly indicate the extent to which mortality may be reduced than a low rate. A sobering thought is that we cannot ignore the specificity rate: the lower this rate is, the greater the number of people who are being unnecessarily disturbed by follow-up procedures to rule out the presence of cancer.

Cost-Effectiveness of Screening

The question of which type of screening is most cost-effective is often asked, usually after efficacy has been established. Costs consist of expenditures in screening a population group, a large majority of whom do not have the disease; follow-up of cases suspicious for cancer; diagnostic tests; and treatment of the cancer. Effectiveness is measured by the reduction of mortality due to the cancer. A criterion for judging cost-effectiveness is needed, and the one advanced for decision-making in medicine has considerable appeal (Doubilet et al., 1986).

One strategy is viewed as more cost-effective than another if it is (1) less costly and at least as effective; (2) more effective and more costly, its additional benefit being worth its additional cost; or (3) less effective and less costly, the added benefit of the rival strategy not being worth its extra cost.

In alternatives 2 and 3, there are three elements (i.e., benefits, costs, and value judgments) that empiricists seek to quantify but that others (e.g., policy-makers, program developers), in many instances, will arrive at on a qualitative basis influenced by more general economic, societal, or political considerations.

Having reached a favorable decision on screening, we have to consider other factors in determining how rapidly screening will spread. Among the more important are the population's health care seeking behaviors, access to care, attitudes, and knowledge, as well as the providers' conviction that screening is indeed effective. Further, organizational and financial characteristics of the delivery system and the nature of its support services can make a difference in how receptive the population is to screening.

Decisions about coverage of screening by nongovernmental health insurance plans affect large segments of the population. Costs are a major consideration but not in a cost-effectiveness context. More important are competitiveness of premiums and attractiveness of new benefits to the consumer; the potential for savings in the long term is too remote to enter significantly into the calculation. This changes, of course, when government mandates inclusion of a specific screening procedure, as has happened in state laws requiring policies to include as a benefit screening for breast cancer with mammography.

> *How different is the situation for reimbursement programs funded by government?*

In this case, inclusion of a service, such as screening, results in a universal entitlement for large groups of people and generates substantial new costs. Clearly, here is an arena where cost-effectiveness might be expected to flourish; advocates of change grapple with cost and effectiveness, while at the same time bringing to bear the weight of societal and political considerations. Within this framework, evidence of benefits from strong research efforts, the RCT, can play a major role.

Methods in Screening

Decision rules have been adopted to link the strength of recommendations for or against a given preventive service (screening) to the quality of the underlying evidence. The Canadian Task Force on the Periodic Health Examination (1979) developed explicit criteria to judge the quality of evidence from published clinical research in the late 1970s. This was followed by a similar effort by the U.S. Preventive Services Task Force, which produced the *Guide to Clinical Preventive Services: An Assessment of the Effectiveness of 169 Interventions* (1989) and, later, an updated, enlarged second edition of the *Guide* (1996).

Study designs

The quality of individual studies was reviewed in connection with each preventive service being considered. Three types of study design received special attention: RCTs, cohort studies, and case-control studies.

RCTs. As noted in the previous chapter on the RCT, randomization increases the comparability of two groups and provides a more valid basis for measuring statistical uncertainty than is true for any other design.

Cohort studies. In a cohort study, the investigators do not determine at the outset which individuals receive the intervention. Individuals are followed longitudinally, to determine the relation between subgroups and outcome. Cohort studies are more subject to systematic bias than RCTs because treatments, risk factors, and other covariables may be chosen by patients or physicians on the basis of factors related to outcome; also important, confounding variables may not be known or be absent from the information available in the study. The disadvantage of both the cohort study and the RCT is that they require large sample sizes and many years of observation.

Case-control studies. The case-control study often avoids some of the problems of the cohort study and the RCT. A detailed discussion of the case-control methodology is found in Chapter 8, but it is worth calling attention to several of its characteristics. The case-control study is retrospective in that cases and controls are selected on the basis of whether they have the adverse outcome; evaluation is designed to determine whether frequency of exposure to the intervention (screening) differs between cases and controls. To the extent that confounding variables can be identified and introduced in the analysis, the case-control methodology is a potent procedure. There may be occasions when it is not possible to carry out an RCT because substantial numbers are already using the intervention. In this case, there is no choice, and the case-control method is an extremely useful substitute study.

Another methodology involves comparisons between a study group of volunteers experiencing the intervention and another group in regular clinical practice. This suffers from the problems of selection of study groups by special characteristics and the inability to take the differences by these characteristics into account. In most cases, the problem is sufficiently severe to prevent drawing even a tentative conclusion regarding the effectiveness of the intervention (screening).

Strength of recommendations for screening

In making judgments regarding the conduct of screening, researchers see considerable overlap between the conditions mentioned earlier in this chapter and the development of the guidelines outlined by the Canadian Task Force on the Periodic Health Examination and the U.S. Preventive Services Task Force. A recommendation for preventive interventions is rated from good to poor; against intervention, it is rated fair or good.

The strength of the recommendation is based on a consideration of three criteria: the burden of suffering from the target condition, the characteristics of the intervention, and the effectiveness of the intervention as demonstrated in published research. Ranking of evidence is as follows:

1. Evidence obtained from at least one properly designed RCT
2.1. Evidence obtained from well-designed trials without randomization

2.2. Evidence obtained from well-designed cohort or case-control analytic studies, preferably from more than one center or research group

2.3. Evidence obtained from multiple time series with or without the intervention

3. Opinions of respected authorities, based on clinical experience, descriptive studies, or reports of expert committees

Screening Studies—Two Case Examples

The screening studies discussed below (breast cancer and colorectal cancer) illustrate the difficulties in reaching conclusions about critical aspects of screening even after many years of research.

Breast cancer screening

Breast cancer has been high on the priority list of cancers for preventive action. An estimated 182,000 cases of newly diagnosed invasive breast cancer are projected for 1995, or about 30% of all cancers detected in the female population of the United States (Wingo et al., 1995). For years, breast cancer was the most common cause of cancer deaths among women. Now, deaths from lung cancer exceed those of breast cancer. This results from a sharp upward trend in mortality from lung cancer rather than a decrease in the breast cancer death rate.

The 5-year relative survival rate among women with breast cancer has been increasing, but the sharp increase in the incidence rate that began during the 1980s has offset this improvement, resulting in a static death rate (except for a very recent decline that may result in part from increased screening) (Ries et al., 1994).

We start the review of trials to test the efficacy of breast cancer screening with a detailed account of a study using the Health Insurance Plan of Greater New York (HIP). This was the first trial conducted, and many of the principles followed in its design were later incorporated in other trials; but there are also fundamental differences among the trials.

The HIP trial. The HIP trial was initiated in 1963 to determine "whether periodic screening with mammography and clinical examination of the breast holds substantial promise for lowering mortality over the long run in the female population from breast cancer" (Shapiro et al., 1988, p. 3). Basic elements of the design and conduct of the trial follow.

Two stratified random samples of women 40–64 years old with at least 1 year's membership in HIP were selected; one group was designated the study group, the other, the control group. The total number of women in each sample was about 31,000, later reduced by about 2%, primarily through the exclusion of women found during the study to have had histologically confirmed breast cancer prior to their entry date.

The efficacy of the screening program was based on changes in measures of mortality due to breast cancer through follow-up of the total study group (i.e., all women scheduled for screening, including those who refused) vs. the control group, ending 18 years from the date of entry.

Women entered the project between December 1963 and June 1966. The screening schedule included an initial examination and three reexaminations at 1-year intervals. About 67% of the study group appeared for initial examinations; high proportions of these women participated in successive cycles of annual examinations. Those in the control group followed their usual practices in obtaining medical care.

Each examination consisted of film mammography (cephalocaudal and lateral views of each breast); a clinical examination of the breast by a physician, usually a surgeon; an interview for demographic and other background information; and a health history. Mammography (two readings by radiologists) and clinical examination of the breast were conducted independently.

To determine whether a woman's underlying cause of death was breast cancer, the death certificate and hospital and physician's records were reviewed; reviewers were blinded to whether the woman was in the experimental or control group.

By 5 years from entry, the numbers of breast cancers detected were very close for total study and control groups (304 and 295, respectively); statements that follow on breast cancers detected are based on these 5-year cases.

Screening resulted in detection of breast cancer at an earlier stage of disease. Breast cancer cases in the total study group (screenees and refusers combined) were more likely to have no histologic evidence of axillary node involvement than control group cases (57% vs. 46%).

Mammography and clinical examinations contributed independently to breast cancer detection. A higher proportion was detected through clinical examination alone than through mammography alone (44.7% vs. 33.3%). The relative contribution of mammography (in the absence of positive clinical findings) was lower among women under 50 years of age (19.4%) than among those 50–59 years (40.9%) and older (31.4%).

The major conclusions regarding efficacy of screening for breast cancer are based on the data for intermediate (10 years from entry) and long-term (18 years from entry) periods of follow-up of cases detected within 5 and 7 years from date of entry. The screening program resulted in about a 30% reduction in mortality from breast cancer during the first 10 years of follow-up in the total study group aged 40–64 years at entry (Table 10-3). By the end of 18 years from entry, the

Table 10-3. Breast cancer deaths among women diagnosed in specified intervals from entry in study and control groups, HIP Trial

| | Number of Breast Cancer Cases[a] | Number of Breast Cancer Deaths Within | |
		10 Years from Entry	18 Years from Entry
Diagnosis 1–5 years after entry			
Study group	307	95	126
Control group	301	133	163
Percent difference		28.6(7.4–45.5)[b]	22.7(2.7–39.0)[b]
Diagnosis 1–7 years after entry			
Study group	431	123	180
Control group	448	174	236
Percent difference		29.3(11.3–44.2)[b]	23.7(7.6–37.4)[b]

[a] Includes deaths among cases histologically confirmed plus deaths among women with breast cancer as the underlying cause but with no histologically confirmed diagnosis before death.

[b] Numbers in parentheses, 95% confidence intervals.

reduction was close to 25%. A favorable effect of screening began to appear appreciably later among women aged 40–49 years at entry than among women above this age. At 18 years from entry, younger women showed a similar reduction in breast cancer mortality; the observation about the level of the difference in breast cancer mortality for women aged 40–49 years at entry has been in dispute with respect to statistical significance.

The differences in timing of the reductions in breast cancer deaths by age at entry might have resulted from a variety of factors: large random variation due to small numbers, relatively low detection of breast cancer among women aged 40–49 years by the mammography available in the 1960s and early 1970s, or an underlying biologic difference in screening's efficacy. Further, a portion of the "benefit" at ages 40–49 years at the time of entry is related to cases detected after women reached 50 years of age.

International studies of screening for breast cancer. A number of RCTs were started in various countries following the release of early data from the HIP trial. In view of the continued controversy regarding the efficacy of screening women at ages 40–49 years, the International Workshop on Screening for Breast Cancer was convened by the National Cancer Institute in 1993 (Fletcher et al., 1993) and, more recently, a consensus development panel (Breast Cancer Screening for Women Ages 40–49, 1997). The meetings reviewed scientific evidence regarding the effectiveness of breast cancer screening, with an emphasis on women aged 40–49 years.

Table 10-4 indicates the high degree of variability in the design and conduct of the trials. In contrast to the HIP trial previously discussed, a Swedish two-

Table 10-4. Characteristics of eight RCTs for breast cancer screening

Study	Screening Modality	Periodicity (months)	% Screened in First Examination
Health Insurance Plan	Two-view MM + CBE	12	67
Sweden			
Two-county	One-view MM	24 (<50 years)	89
		33 (≥50 years)	
Malmo	Two-view MM	18–24	74
Stockholm	One-view MM	28	81
Gothenburg	Two-view MM	18	84
Edinburgh, Scotland	CBE	12	61
	Two-view MM initial, later one-view	24	
Canada			
40–49 years	Two-view MM + CBE	12	100
50–59 years	Two-view MM + CBE vs. CBE only	12	100

MM, mammography; CBE, clinical breast examination.

Source: Fletcher et al. (1993).

county trial sampled geographic clusters and used single-view mammography at 24-month intervals (ages 40–49 years) and 33-month intervals (ages 50–74 years); 89% attended the first screening. Two trials, Edinburgh, Scotland, and Malmo, Sweden, started at age 45 years. In the Canadian National Breast Screening Study, volunteers were recruited for randomized allocation to study and control groups. At ages 40–49 years, study women had an initial screening and three or four rescreenings with clinical breast examination (CBE) and two-view mammography; control women had only a CBE at the initial screening. At ages 50–59 years, CBE and two-view mammography were available for four or five screenings (study group). CBE was offered to the control group in each round of screening, and the trial in this age group aimed at determining the value of adding mammography to CBE under screening conditions.

Table 10-5 shows a high degree of consistency among the trials in the reduction of breast cancer mortality for the study group of women who were offered screening. The overall decrease was in the range of 25–30%. All trials have examined data by age subgroups, but in each case, the samples had low statistical power to find even large differences if they existed. Variations in the design and conduct of the trials have been cited as additional reasons for not accepting the results related to women aged 40–49 years. Nonetheless, it was speculated that if a pattern emerged across studies, confidence would increase in drawing conclusions about the effectiveness of screening.

The result for women aged 40–49 years in the HIP trial has already been

Table 10-5. Age at entry, duration of follow-up, and relative risk for deaths due to breast cancer in study group vs. control group (all ages)

Trial	Age at Entry (Years)	Follow-Up (Years)	Relative Risk
Health Insurance Plan[a]	40–64	10	0.71 (0.55–0.93)[b]
Sweden			
Kopparberg[c]	40–74	12	0.68 (0.52–0.89)
Ostergotland[c]	40–74	12	0.82 (0.64–1.05)
Malmo	45–69	12	0.81 (0.62–1.07)
Stockholm	40–64	8	0.80 (0.53–1.22)
Gothenburg	40–59	7	0.86 (0.54–1.37)
All centers	40–74	7–12	0.76 (0.66–0.87)
Edinburg, Scotland	45–64	10	0.84 (0.63–1.12)
Canada[d]	50–59	7	0.97 (0.62–1.52)

[a]Eighteen years from entry: relative risk = 0.77 (95% confidence interval 0.61–0.97).

[b]Numbers in parentheses, 95% confidence interval.

[c]Two-county Swedish trial.

[d]Comparison is between mammography plus clinical breast examination vs. clinical breast examination alone.

Source: Fletcher et al. (1993).

discussed. Table 10-6 gives data from all RCTs that have been carried out. In the Swedish trials, one county, Kopparberg, showed a large favorable outcome (relative risk = 0.67); the other county, Ostergotland, showed a relative risk of 1.02. In Malmo, the only other area with a long period of follow-up, the relative risk was low at ages 45–49 years. When the trials in Sweden are combined, there is an observed decrease in mortality of 23% in women aged 40–49 years in the study group (95% confidence interval [CI] 0.59–1.01) (Nystrom et al., 1997).

A nonstatistically significant relative risk of 0.88 (95% CI 0.55–1.41) was found in the Edinburgh trial for women 45–49 years old at 14 years; in the Canadian trial, the relative risk was in the opposite direction at 10 years (1.14, 95% CI 0.83–1.56), and a longer period of follow-up is needed.

The report on the workshop in 1993 concluded that RCTs consistent in showing no benefit in breast cancer mortality for women aged 40–49 years at 5–7 years after entry and an uncertain and, if present, marginal benefit at 10–12 years; more information is needed before firm conclusions can be drawn about any delayed effects of screening on mortality. The 1997 consensus development conference agreed with the conclusion that benefit among women aged 40–49 years when screening started was not established (Breast Cancer Screening for Women Ages 40–49, 1997). However, the National Cancer Institute accepted the recommendation from the National Cancer Advisory Board to include women aged 40–49 years in routine screening programs.

Convincing evidence for the benefit of mammographic screening has been

Table 10-6. Relative risk for deaths due to breast cancer in study group vs. control group in RCTs (aged 40–49 years at entry)

Trial	Follow-Up (Years)	Relative Risk
Health Insurance Plan[a]	10	0.77 (0.50–1.16)[b]
Sweden		
Kopparberg[c]	17	0.67 (0.37–1.22)
Ostergotland[c]	16	1.02 (0.59–1.77)
Malmo	17	0.67 (0.35–1.27)
Stockholm	13	1.34 (0.64–2.50)
Gothenburg	10	0.59 (0.33–1.06)
All centers	17[e]	0.77 (0.59–1.01)
Edinburgh, Scotland	14	0.88 (0.55–1.41)
Canada[d]	10	1.14 (0.83–1.56)

[a]Eighteen years from entry: relative risk = 0.77 (95% confidence interval 0.61–0.97).

[b]Numbers in parentheses, 95% confidence intervals.

[c]Two-county Swedish trial.

[d]Comparison is between mammography plus clinical breast examination vs. clinical breast examination alone at initial screening; subsequently, no examination.

[e]Upper limits used for all Swedish trials.

Source: Fletcher et al. (1993), Nystrom et al. (1997).

shown for women aged 50–69 years (Table 10-7). In all studies, the relative risk was lower for study groups of women in this age range and started much earlier than among women aged 40–49 years. The decrease in breast cancer mortality is about 30%. This finding holds true despite the fact that only the Swedish two-county and HIP studies resulted in statistically significant differentials in relative risk.

There is no research to determine whether an age threshold exists beyond which screening ceases to be of benefit. However, the National Institutes of Health Breast Cancer Screening Forum (Costanza et al., 1992) urged that considerations about screening older women be based on a woman's general health and that decisions regarding screening should be made jointly by the woman and her physician and should reflect her comorbidity. This position is taken primarily because of the substantially higher risk of breast cancer in women at these ages and their increased life expectancy.

Comment. Critics of the conclusion that there is uncertainty regarding the efficacy of mammography screening at ages 40–49 years (Kopans et al., 1994; Sickles and Kopans, 1995) have emphasized that these trials, except for the Canadian study, were not designed to assess the efficacy of screening at particular ages. None has statistical power to detect meaningful benefits by age. Other criticisms have been aimed at the trials' conduct, which affects results for women

Table 10-7. Relative risk for deaths due to breast cancer in study group vs. control group: Health Insurance Plan (HIP), Sweden, and Edinburgh, Scotland (aged 50 years and older at entry)

Trial	Relative Risk
HIP (10 years), 50–64 years old	0.68 (0.49–0.96)[a]
Swedish centers combined (12 years)[b]	
50–59 years old	0.71 (0.57–0.90)
60–69 years old	0.71 (0.56–0.91)
70–74 years old	0.94 (0.60–1.46)
Edinburg (10 years), 50–64 years old[b]	0.85 (0.63–1.46)

[a] Numbers in parentheses, 95% confidence intervals.

[b] Data presented at International Workshop on Screening for Breast Cancer, February 24–25, 1993.

Source: Fletcher et al. (1993).

aged 40–49 years. In the Canadian study, the issues cited were poor quality of mammography in the early years and possible aberrations in the sampling procedure. Problems with the Swedish two-county trial included the use of single-view mammography and a 2-year interval of screening at the ages of 40–49 years. More generally, statistical power was reduced in most, if not all, of the trials owing to the use of mammography by some women in the control group.

There are counterarguments (Baines, 1994; Shapiro, 1994). For example, crossover by controls does not come close to the far greater exposure to screening mammography in the intervention group, and the Canadian trials demonstrate that mammography had made substantial contributions in the detection of breast cancer. In the end, a choice has to be made about the evidence with regard to screening women aged 40–49 years: either to conclude that the results of the trials are too uncertain to support mass mammography screening as a public health measure or to reject the studies, individually or collectively, as inadequate. In either case, there is no scientific support for a public health policy that advocates routine screening of women aged 40–49 years with mammography (i.e., a policy that actively encourages all asymptomatic women to seek screening with mammography).

In most countries, the policies for breast cancer screening exclude women under 50 years of age, provide for screening at longer routine intervals than annually, have two views of mammography only for the initial screening examination, and do not include the physical examination as part of screening. The American Cancer Society's guidelines promote routine screening with mammography at annual intervals for women aged 40–49 years as well as women aged

50 years and older; CBEs are to be performed annually. The National Cancer Institute calls attention to the controversy about routine screening mammography at the ages of 40–49 years and indicates that routine screening every 1 or 2 years with mammography can reduce breast cancer mortality for women aged 40–49 as well as those aged 50 years and over. Emphasis is given to the need for a CBE by a health care provider in regular, routine health care.

Several actions are being taken to settle the issue concerning the value of screening with mammography at ages under 50 years. The most ambitious is the initiation of a new trial in the United Kingdom in which women aged 40–41 years are invited to have an annual mammography screening. The reason for the restriction of screening to the 40–41-year age group is to avoid the problem demonstrated in the HIP trial. Here, part of the gain found among women aged 40–49 years at the time of entry was concentrated in the subgroup who had passed their fiftieth birthday when breast cancer was detected during the screening program. In the United Kingdom trial, all women will be eligible for screening at the age of 50 years, and the test will be to see how much benefit is obtained by starting to screen women in their forties. Additional years of experience are being gained in the studies started some time ago, and these are to be examined for new insights on whether screening younger women is efficacious.

Based on the material presented, what would be a reasonable appraisal of the questions raised below?

Each has been the subject of many commentaries. The one that has been presented above is usually favored by epidemiologists and family practitioners, but criticisms have been advanced by voluntary health agencies, lay advocates for promoting routine screening, and radiologists. In answering the questions, the reader must often choose between two positions, which is best taken up in a group discussion.

1. Can we learn anything from the age-specific results of the studies, or should we set them aside and concentrate on the overall results?
2. What have we gained through the conduct of multiple trials in determining the value of routine breast cancer screening?
3. Should the Canadian trial be included in an overview analysis of the value of routine screening of women aged 40–49 years? (The question arises because of the criticisms of the trial and the relatively short duration of follow-up—thus far, 10 years.)
4. How do you appraise the recommendation of the National Cancer Institute that screening women aged 40–49 years should be routine?

Colorectal cancer screening

Colorectal cancer is the fourth most frequently diagnosed cancer annually, being exceeded by cancers of the lung, breast, and prostate (Wingo et al., 1995). In terms of mortality, it is second only to lung cancer. It was estimated that for 1995 138,200 new cases of colorectal cancer would be diagnosed and that 55,300 would die from this condition. The incidence is increasing, but the mortality is decreasing. The incidence is higher in men than in women (60.4 vs. 40.9/100,000 years); the rate increases sharply after the age of 50 years.

Status of studies of the effectiveness of screening for colorectal cancer. Toward the end of the 1960s, fecal occult blood testing was developed for early detection of the condition; later, other advances included use of the flexible sigmoidoscope and diagnostic colonoscopy. A number of studies designed to detect colorectal cancer at an earlier stage than is found in clinical practice have been carried out (or are still under way) in the hope that this would lead to lowered mortality. Several of the studies showed very favorable results using the sigmoidoscope, but, until recently, they did not have comparison groups.

Two case-control studies that evaluate the effectiveness of screening sigmoidoscopy in preventing colorectal cancer mortality have been reported (Newcomb et al., 1992; Selby et al., 1992). Both were conducted in prepaid health plans. Rigid sigmoidoscopy was applied during the period evaluated by Selby et al. (1992); rigid and flexible sigmoidoscopic examinations were used in the study by Newcomb et al. (1992). Both studies suggested a significantly decreased risk (60–80%) of fatal cancer of the distal colon or rectum among individuals with a history of one or more sigmoidoscopic examinations compared with nonscreened patients. These studies have been interpreted differently. On the one hand, they are seen as providing proof of the strong efficacious value of screening with sigmoidoscopy. On the other hand, it is argued that they do not establish efficacy because of the possibility of biases. The National Cancer Institute has initiated a randomized trial of the efficacy of periodic examinations with a flexible sigmoidoscope among individuals aged 60–74 years (baseline and another screening 3 years later).

> *Should the results of the case-control studies be viewed as promising or as proof that screening with flexible sigmoidoscopy leads to a reduction in colorectal cancer?*

RCTs to test the efficacy of screening for colorectal cancer. Five RCTs are under way to evaluate the efficacy of periodic screening for colorectal cancer utilizing the fecal occult blood test. A trial in Sweden is aimed at individuals aged 60–64 years (Kewenter et al., 1988). A study in England provides screening to candidates drawn from lists of family practitioners (Harcastle et al., 1989). A Danish trial offers screening to individuals aged 45–75 years, allocated at random to a control and a study group (Kronborg et al., 1989). The Memorial Sloan-Kettering Cancer Center-Strang Clinic trial was an evaluation of the fecal occult blood test as a supplement to annual rigid sigmoidoscopy (Winawer et al., 1993). The only RCT that has produced definitive results thus far is the Minnesota Colon Cancer Control Study. The balance of this discussion concentrates on the methods used and the findings of this study (Mandel et al., 1993).

From 1975 through 1977, 46,551 volunteers, aged 50–80 years, were recruited from various organizations and employee groups in Minnesota; criteria were established for exclusion of individuals with a history of colorectal cancer, familial polyposis, and other conditions. Volunteers were stratified by age, sex, and place of residence and then randomly assigned to screening once a year or once every 2 years or to a control group that continued to receive their usual medical care. The intervention consisted of six guaiac-impregnated paper slides (Hemoccult); the slides contained two smears from each of three consecutive stools, and each slide was rehydrated starting in 1977. Patients with one or more slides testing positive were asked to appear at the hospital for diagnostic workup. Colonoscopy was administered throughout the study, with biopsies of visible lesions performed; all substantial abnormalities, particularly polyps and cancers, were treated.

Participants in all three study groups were mailed questionnaires annually to determine their vital status, the occurrence of colorectal cancer and polyps in the control group, and similar information from the screened groups for diagnoses not due to the screening examinations. Death certificates were obtained for virtually all patients who died; the death records along with medical records were reviewed. Reviewers were blinded concerning the study status of the deceased, to arrive at the underlying cause of death.

It was planned to screen the participants for 5 years and to follow them for an additional 5 years, with the screening phase to end in 1982. This was later changed, and screening was resumed from 1986 until 1992. The reason was that mortality from colorectal cancer was lower than had been estimated at the start of the study, when the power calculations were carried out for sample size.

The annually screened group completed 75.2% of the screening examinations, and the biennially screened group completed 78.4%. Almost half (46.2%) of the former group completed all of the screenings; this compares with 59.2% of the biennial group. A large majority (75%) of the screened group with positive findings were further examined at the University of Minnesota Hospital, with over 96% undergoing colonoscopy. Of those with a positive fecal occult blood test examined elsewhere, 44% had a colonoscopy and 42% had a flexible sigmoidoscopy and barium enema but no colonoscopy.

The cumulative incidence of colorectal cancer was very similar in the three groups; the cumulative annual mortality rate for colorectal cancer was lower in the annually screened group (5.88/1,000) than in the biennially screened group (8.33/1,000) and the control group (8.83/1,000) (Table 10-8). The relative risk for colorectal cancer was 0.67 (95% CI 0.50–0.87), annual vs. control; the relative risk was not statistically significant between the biennial and control groups (0.94, 95% CI 0.68–1.31). Adjustments for age, sex, and place of residence by Cox proportional hazards regression did not alter the statistically significant difference in relative risks between the annual screening group and the controls.

Changes in the incidence of Dukes' stages were consistent with the findings in mortality from colorectal cancer (Table 10-9). Stages A and B had a higher incidence in the screened groups; stage D was found almost twice as often in the control group as in the annually screened group (4.4 and 2.3/1,000, respectively). Survival at 5 years was only 2.4% for patients with Dukes' stage D cancers; survival ranged from 94.3% (stage A) to 56.6% (stage C) in the 13 years of follow-up.

Rehydration played an important role in the cancer screening. The rate of positive results increased from 2.4% to 9.8% when rehydration became routine (Table 10-10). Rehydration increased the sensitivity of the screening from 80.8% to 92.2% and decreased the specificity from 97.7% to 90.4%; the positive predictive value decreased from 5.6% to 2.2%.

Comment. This is the first RCT that has shown a benefit from screening with fecal occult blood tests. The 33% reduction in the colorectal cancer death rate in the annually screened group was statistically significant; the 6% decrease in the biennially screened group was not, and additional follow-up is needed to settle the issue about the value of screening less frequently than annually.

About 85% of the slides were rehydrated, increasing incidence rates and the frequency of colonoscopies, but the specificity rate decreased.

During the first 8 years of follow-up, the incidence rates for colorectal cancer were about the same in the three groups in the study; during the next 5 years, the incidence rates in the screened groups were lower than that in the control group.

The positive results of this trial have strengthened the position of advocates of the fecal occult blood test, but there are others who have reservations about the strength of the trial in promoting screening. The questions that follow represent several of the more important that have been raised. They demonstrate that no single RCT can answer all of the questions that arise.

Table 10-8. Mortality and incidence of colorectal cancer per 1,000, according to study group, during the 13 years after randomization

Study Group	Persons-Years in the Study	Colorectal Cancer		Deaths from All Cancers		Deaths from Colorectal Cancer		
		Number of Cases	Cumulative Incidence[a]	Number of Deaths	Cumulative Mortality[a]	Number of Deaths	Cumulative Mortality[a]	Cumulative Mortality Ratio
Annual Screening	184,160	323	23 (21–26)[b]	3,361	216 (209–222)[b]	82	5.88 (4.61–7.15)	0.67 (0.50–0.87)[c]
Biennial screening	183,934	323	23 (20–25)	3,396	218 (211–224)	117	8.33 (6.82–9.84)	0.94 (0.68–1.31)
Control	181,966	356	26 (23–28)	3,340	216 (210–223)	121	8.83 (7.26–10.40)	1.00

[a]Numbers of deaths from colorectal cancer are based on determinations by the Deaths Review Committee.

[b]Numbers in parentheses, 95% confidence intervals.

[c]Adjusted for sequential monitoring.

Table 10-9. Colorectal cancers, according to study group and Dukes' stage, and 5-year survival according to stage

| | Number of Cancers by Study Group | | | | |
Stage	Annual Screening	Biennial Screening	Control	All	5-Year Survival (%)
A	107	98	88	293	94.3
B	101	95	120	316	84.4
C	80	100	82	262	56.6
D	33	41	65	139	2.4
Unstaged	33	34	39	106	87.0
All	354	368	394	1,116	70.0

1. How important are the increase in sensitivity and the decrease in specificity in deciding whether to launch a national campaign with the fecal occult blood test?
2. Does the high proportion of study women with a positive fecal occult blood test who had a colonoscopy, a costly procedure, affect the interpretation of the value of the former test?
3. Does the trial prevent colorectal cancer because of the removal of polyps?
4. Is there any evidence in the reported material that supports a reduction in incidence?

The possibility that the control group may have participated in fecal occult blood testing and thereby reduced the effect of the screening program has been raised. However, with only 1.8% of the colorectal cases in the control group associated with such tests, this factor can be dismissed. Another issue is whether a larger proportion of the screened groups had received treatment for colorectal cancer at the University of Minnesota Hospital than the control group (22% vs.

Table 10-10. Positivity, sensitivity, specificity, and positive predictive value of testing for colorectal cancer, according to rehydration status of slides, in both screening groups combined[a]

	Positivity	Sensitivity[b]	Specificity[c]	Positive Predictive Value (%)[d]
Rehydration	9.8	92.2	90.4	2.2
No rehydration	2.4	80.8	97.7	5.6

[a] Data are based an results from 1976 through 1982.

[b] Sensitivity is the number of true-positive results divided by the sum of true-positive results and true-negative results.

[c] Specificity is the number of true-negative results divided by the sum of true-negatives and false-positives.

[d] Positive predictive values are true-positive results divided by the sum of true-positives and false-positives.

very few) and thereby caused a spurious difference in survival. Additional follow-up is being carried out to investigate whether a decrease in colorectal cancer death rates will appear between the subjects scheduled for screening biennially and the controls.

Conclusion

Two cancer sites in which screening has been advanced as a procedure that could lead to a reduction in mortality have been discussed in this chapter. For each site, there is general agreement that the strongest evidence for formulating a policy that advocates screening needs to come from positive results of RCTs. The rationale for this position is based on several factors: screening is costly since, by definition, it is aimed at the total population at risk, but the incidence of the disease is relatively low; unnecessary procedures are performed because of false-positive findings in screening; and cancers are diagnosed that may never appear clinically.

The most persuasive evidence that screening's benefits outweigh the risks and costs would come from the results of multiple trials with similar designs. In the case of breast cancer screening, we come closest to meeting this objective. Multiple trials have been conducted, but these have varied as to whether or not a CBE was included in the screening examination, the periodicity of screening, and the age groups targeted. However, the fact that the trials show similar findings about the value of screening has stimulated many countries to introduce screening. It is clear that positive results can be achieved in programs that are designed differently. The one issue on which there is disagreement in the United States concerns the age at which to start screening. Further study is needed on the value of starting to screen women at the ages of 40–49 years.

Colorectal screening with fecal occult blood testing has been confirmed as a useful technique through the results of annual testing in the Minnesota RCT. Other tests are being conducted in Europe, but it is not certain when data will be available. Questions are being raised about the costs of the rehydration method used, the loss in specificity that occurs, and the possibility that the fecal occult blood test is really a screening method to identify patients who should have a colonoscopy. The frequency of colonoscopy, over 90% of those with a positive fecal occult blood test who have follow-up examinations at the Minnesota Hospital, is a significant issue. With longer follow-up, it would be possible to determine whether colonoscopy serves an additional function, that is, reducing the incidence of colorectal cancer through the removal of polyps.

The results of two case-control studies have focused attention on the likelihood that sigmoidoscopy might be an effective routine screening procedure for the reduction of colorectal cancer. The National Cancer Institute has an RCT under way on the efficacy of administering flexible sigmoidoscopy twice, at baseline and 3 years later. As matters stand now, we have an example in which an RCT has demonstrated that it is possible to change the natural history of colorectal cancer through screening with a fecal occult blood test and follow-up of positive cases with colonoscopy.

What emerges from the discussion of breast and colorectal cancer screening is the primacy of RCTs in reaching a decision that affects the general population. Questions that agitate the relevant field of patients and providers of care remain outstanding, but we can speak more authoritatively about the power of the results of the trials than if we were dependent on clinical or observational studies or mathematical modeling. This is seen in connection with prostate cancer screening, where no RCT has been completed, but many studies have been conducted to refine the criteria for making a judgment about the likelihood that prostate cancer is present. The measure that has been most intensively investigated in recent years is the prostate-specific antigen, which detects prostate cancer early, but the extent to which cases are being detected that would ordinarily never be seen in clinical practice and whether the measure should become part of routine screening are not known.

References

Baines, C. J. 1994. A different view on what is known about breast screening and the Canadian National Breast Screening Study. *Cancer,* 74:1207–1211.

Breast Cancer Screening for Women Ages 40–49. NIH Concensus Development Statement 1997; 15(1) in press.

Canadian Task Force on the Periodic Health Examination. 1979. The periodic health examination. *Can. Med. Assoc. J.,* 121:1193–1254.

Costanza, M. E., G. J. Annas, M. L. Brown, et al. 1992. Supporting statements and rationale. *J. Gerontol.,* 47:7–16.

Doubilet, P., M. C. Weinstein, and B. J. McNeil. 1986. Use and misuse of the term ''cost effective'' in medicine. *N. Engl. J. Med.,* 314:253–256.

Fletcher, S. W., W. Black, R. Harris, et al. 1993. Special article: report of the International Workshop on Screening for Breast Cancer. *J. Natl. Cancer Inst.,* 85:1644–1656.

Harcastle, J. D., J. D. Thomas, J. Chamberlain, et al. 1989. Randomized controlled trial of faecal occult blood screening for colorectal cancer; results for first 107349 subjects. *Lancet,* i:1160–1164.

Kewenter, J., S. Bjork, E. Haglind, et al. 1988. Screening and rescreening for colorectal cancer: a controlled trial of fecal occult blood testing in 27,700 subjects. *Cancer,* 62:645–651.

Kopans, D. B., E. Halpern, and C. A. Hulka. 1994. Statistical power in breast cancer screening trials and mortality reduction among women 40–49 years of age with particular emphasis on the National Breast Screening Study of Canada. *Cancer,* 74:1196–1203.

Kronborg, O., C. Fenger, J. Olsen, et al. 1989. Repeated screening for colorectal cancer with fecal occult blood test: a prospective randomized study at Funen, Denmark. *Scand. J. Gastroenterol.*, 24:599–606.

Mandel, J. S., J. H. Bond, T. R. Church, et al. 1993. Reducing mortality from colorectal cancer by screening for fecal occult blood. *N. Engl. J. Med.*, 328:1365–1371.

Newcomb, P. A., R. G. Norfleet, B. E. Storer, et al. 1992. Screening sigmoidoscopy and colorectal cancer mortality. *J. Natl. Cancer Inst.*, 84:1572–1575.

Nystrom, L., S. Wall, L. E. Rutqvist, et al. 1997. Update of the overview of the Swedish randomized trials on breast cancer screening with mammography. NIH Consensus Development Conference.

Ries, L. A. G., B. A. Miller, B. F. Hankey, et al., eds. 1994. *SEER Cancer Statistics Review, 1973–1991*. Bethesda, MD: National Cancer Institute.

Selby, J., G. E. Friedman, C. P. Quesenberry, Jr., et al. 1992. A case-control study of screening sigmoidoscopy and mortality from colorectal cancer. *N. Engl. J. Med.*, 326:653–657.

Shapiro, S. 1994. The call for change in breast cancer screening guidelines. *Am. J. Public Health*, 84:10–11.

Shapiro, S., W. Venet, P. Strax, et al. 1988. *Periodic Screening For Breast Cancer, The Health Insurance Plan Project and Its Sequelae, 1963-1986*. Baltimore: Johns Hopkins University Press.

Sickles, E. A., and D. B. Kopans. 1995. Mammographic screening for women aged 40 to 49 years: the primary care practitioner's dilemma. *Ann. Intern. Med.*, 122:534–538.

U.S. Preventive Services Task Force. 1989. *Guide to Clinical Preventive Services: An Assessment of the Effectiveness of 169 Interventions*. Baltimore: Williams & Wilkins.

U.S. Preventive Services Task Force. 1996. *Guide to Clinical Preventive Services*, 2nd ed. Baltimore: Williams & Wilkins.

Wilson, J., and G. Jungren. 1968. *Principles and Practice of Screening for Disease*. Geneva: World Health Organization.

Winawer, S. J., B. J. Flehinger, D. Schottenfeld, et al. 1993. Screening for colorectal cancer with fecal occult blood testing and sigmoidoscopy. *J. Natl. Cancer Inst.*, 85:1311–1318.

Wingo, P. A., T. Tong, and S. Bolden. 1995. Cancer statistics, 1995. *CA Cancer J. Clin.*, 45:8–30.

CHAPTER 11

Analytic
Approaches

DONALD R. HOOVER

This chapter illustrates the application of analytic (statistical) methods to epidemiologic research on a major health service problem: drug use and human immunodeficiency virus (HIV) infection. It begins with an evaluation of case studies that originally drew this problem to the attention of the medical community and progresses to intervention trials that set the stage for program development. The analytic methods for the epidemiologic research described in this chapter can be applied to other problems in health services and policy.

The biologic, medical, and economic context of a health services program defines the context within which epidemiologic research and the corresponding analytic methods will be performed. HIV is transmitted from person to person and leads to acquired immune deficiency syndrome (AIDS) and death. The causal organism (HIV) apparently entered the American population in the late 1970s, and the disease was recognized at the end of 1980 (Shilts, 1987). This disease has a very long incubation period (~10 years) (Merrigan and Balognesi, 1993), and the early stage of infection is silent, making it difficult to identify infected individuals in order to treat the disease palliatively or prevent further transmission. There is still no cure for HIV type 1 (HIV-1) disease nor does a successful vaccine appear imminent. The end-stage opportunistic infections and malignant diseases associated with AIDS are difficult to manage and thus put a heavy burden on the health care system (Merrigan and Balognesi, 1993).

The only current avenue to reduce the burden of HIV disease it to identify and eliminate activities that promote person-to-person spread of the causal organism. This chapter describes a progressive series of epidemiologic investigations leading toward this public health goal and the corresponding analytic methods. It is organized according to the chronologic order of the types of study being conductd, starting with case investigations that identify a specific person-to-person mode of HIV transmission and ending with intervention studies and proposals for health services program development. The statistical research tools needed to implement the epidemiologic methods described in the previous chapters as well as additional statistical approaches are illustrated in the examples.

Case Investigations

As described in Chapter 7, the initial step in studying a health services problem is the case investigations that identify the problem. For HIV-1 disease and AIDS, homosexual men were the first group to be recognized as being at risk. Soon afterward, injection drug users were identified as a risk group. These early inferences were based on case studies reported in the medical literature. Detailed initial case reports of AIDS among drug users can be found in the literature (Merrigan and Balognesi, 1993). Below is a condensed hypothetical example of how an early case study of HIV-1 disease in an injection drug user would be reported.

> In 1982, Miss R. was diagnosed with *Pneumocystis carinii* pneumonia and cytomegalovirus disease, both AIDS-related illnesses previously identified among homosexual men. A blood test revealed that Miss R. had CD4 lymphocyte counts of 50/μl. Homosexual AIDS case patients also had reduced CD4 counts in this range, compared with 1,000/μl for healthy individuals.
>
> Previously, sexual activities with an infected bisexual male partner were thought to be the only mechanism for transmission of the causal agent of AIDS to women, but Miss R. reported having no sexual contact with a man for over 5 years. She did, however, have a friend, Mrs. S., whose husband was bisexual. Furthermore, Miss R. and Mrs. S. regualrly injected cocaine together and shared needles. The process of sharing needles results in sharing residual blood that gets sucked into the needle after each injection and then pushed out into the veins of the next injectee. Mrs. S. also had an 18-month-old child who had died of *P. carinii* pneumonia recently.

Questions:
1. What is the purpose of case investigations such as this?
2. What is the key hypothesis that the above report raises?
3. What are the analytic methods used in this case investigation?
4. What other information should the investigators have obtained and reported for the above case study?
5. Based on this case report, what other approaches should be taken to ascertain the role of shared needles in HIV-1 disease and its medical significance?

Case-Control and Cross-Sectional Studies

Early in the HIV epidemic, numerous AIDS cases were identified among different intravenous drug users who shared needles (Merrigan and Balognesi, 1993;

Normand et al., 1995). AIDS cases were also identified in children who were vaccinated with a shared needle. In addition, transmission of other pathogens through blood contact has been well established (Benenson, 1995). In spite of all this evidence, a direct conclusion of blood-borne transmission of HIV through shared needles cannot be reached without further investigation. It cannot be ruled out that other factors associated with injection drug use (e.g., noninjection drug use and promiscuous sex) are responsible for HIV infection and AIDS. Injection drug users could be more sexually active than the rest of the population and contracting HIV through sex. Given the importance of this problem and the implications for health intervention, well-designed epidemiologic investigations are needed to determine that needle sharing does (or does not) cause transmission of the causal agent for AIDS.

The initial studies usually performed to resolve the question of causality raised by early case studies and illustrated in Figure 11-1, are case-control (Chapter 8) or cross-sectional (Chapter 5). Within such studies, competing mechanisms of causality are explored by examining groups of individuals with diverse attributes or behaviors that can separate out the potential impacts of competing mechanisms.

Question:
6. Why are population follow-up studies or clinical trials usually not the first epidemiologic investigations performed, rather than case-control or cross-sectional studies?

We now illustrate how a case-control study of this issue would be conducted. An immunologist, Dr. M., believes that HIV is actually being spread through sexual contact among drug users. He has observed that a specific human immunity function is lowered after repeated injections of drugs. He believes this lowered immunity makes these individuals more susceptible to HIV infection for sexual contact and that shared blood itself does not contribute to transmission. He noted that spiked injections of external insulin restore this immunity function in drug users. He also observed that illicit drug users who are diabetics (and thus inject insulin regularly) did not have this lowered immunity function, while other injection drug users always did.

He plans to study this hypothesized protective effect of insulin by making a comparison of rates of diabetes among drug users who test positive for HIV (cases) and those who test negative for HIV (controls). (A serologic blood test is available that can test for HIV infection.) If the HIV-infected drug user group has less diabetics than the noninfected drug user group, this might support Dr. M.'s hypothesis that insulin use counters HIV transmission among drug users and provides a potential mechanism to stop the spread of HIV.

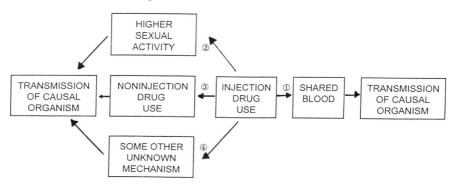

Route ① was postulated in the case studies described in the text
Route ②, ③ and ④ are other potential mechanisms

Figure 11-1. Potential causes of HIV/AIDS among injection drug users identified in case studies.

Power and Sample Size

Whenever an investigation is undertaken that requires commitment of time and resources, the researchers need to be certian that the study has a sufficient chance to prove the hypothesis of interest. This is analogous to studying the cost-effectiveness of implementation of programs in economics and is referred to in the field of statistics as "power" analysis. The issue of power is important in not only case control studies but also, as was discussed in Chapters 6 and 9, in cross-sectional studies, population studies, and clinical trials.

Various statistical approaches have been developed to explore the potential power of a planned study (cf., Fleiss, 1981; Shuster, 1990). While the statistical details of these approaches are beyond the scope of this chapter, health researchers often will collaborate with statisticians to estimate the power of a proposed study. Thus, it is important to understand the concepts behind power and sample size analysis.

Typically, a study compares two groups of individuals (exposed and unexposed) to see if an outcome of interest occurs more (or less) in the exposed group than in the unexposed group. For example, in Dr. M.'s study, the exposure is external insulin injection for diabetes (yes/no) and the outcome is HIV-1 infection. Because the occurrence of HIV infection is random, not deterministic, it is possible by chance that HIV infection would not be more common in the non-diabetic group than in the insulin injecting diabetic group, even if insulin injection protects against HIV infection.

A failure to statistically reject the null hypothesis of equal occurrence of outcome in both groups (exposed/unexposed), when the null hypothesis is truly false, is called a β-error. Conversely, the power, or the chance to reject the null hypothesis when it is false, is $1 - \beta$. The chance for a β-error to occur depends on how false the null hypothesis is. If (i) insulin injecting diabetics are only slightly less likely to contract HIV infection than are nondiabetics, then a study is more likely to fail to detect a difference than if (ii) diabetics are much less likely to contract HIV infection than are nondiabetics. Thus, to define the β-error, the investigator must be able either to estimate how large the difference in HIV infection between diabetics and nondiabetics is likely to be from preliminary data or to know how large the true difference needs to be to have medical importance.

Conversely, it is possible to falsely reject the null hypothesis when, in fact, it is true (i.e., no real difference between diabetics and nondiabetics exists). This occurs because, by chance alone, the outcome could occur more in one group than in the other and is called an α-error.

For any given study conducted, the chances of making either an α-error or a β-error range between 0 and 1 (0–100%). The investigator would like to conduct a study that simultaneously has low chances of making α- and β-errors. Typically, the investigator sets the α-error at 0.05, only a 5% chance to reject the null hypothesis when it is true. A β-error of less than 0.20 (only a 20% chance to not reject the null hypothesis if it is false) is usually desired. Thus, the investigator tries to design a study that has α- and β-errors at least as low as 0.05 and 0.20, respectively.

Everything being equal, larger studies with more subjects have lower α- and β-errors than do smaller studies. However, larger studies are more expensive, and sometimes the total number of potential participants may be limited. For a given number of cases and controls, expected true probabilities for exposure in each group under the null and alternative hypotheses, and a a set α-error, statistical formulas exist to calculate the β-error of the study (Fleiss, 1981). These formulas also can be used to estimate the minimal number of cases and controls needed for a study to have given α- and β-errors. The formulas can be implemented by several software packages with the help of a statistician.

For example, in the case-control study of Dr. M., let $n_1 = 400$ HIV$^-$ intravenous drug user controls and let $n_2 = 200$ HIV$^+$ intravenous drug user cases, setting the α-error to 0.05. Assume that $P_1 = 10\%$ of the population of drug users in a given area are insulin injecting diabetics, and, it is believed, based on reports from elsewhere, that $P_2 = 5\%$ of diabetic drug users are infected with HIV-1. Then, based on a statistical formula from Fleiss (1981), the β-error of this study will be 0.42. If this same study were conducted 100 times, about 42 of these times it would fail to find a different rate of HIV infection in diabetic and nondiabetic drug users when, in fact, 10% of nondiabetics and 5% of diabetics in the entire population were infected with HIV. The power of the study is $1 - \beta$, or, in this case, 0.58. If the investigator wishes to lower the β-error to 0.20 and increase the power to 0.80, the sample sizes n_1 and/or n_2 must be increased.

While the issue of power and sample size is important, it has been covered only briefly here. To be good, a study must be able to use the available data (the n_1 controls and n_2 cases) to have a high probability (power) to detect a reasonable alternative hypothesis (when it is true) while simultaneously having a low probability to reject the null hypothesis (α-error) when it is true. When fitting power formulas to population-based studies (Chapter 5) and clinical trials (Chapter 9), n_1 would be the number exposed and n_2 would be the number not exposed.

Remember the importance of this issue when planning studies and be prepared to consult with a statistician if needed. In addition, the numbers the statistician inputs into the formula, P_1, P_2, n_1 and n_2, as well as α, must be chosen carefully and judiciously based on the best available data. Judgment is involved, and an important decision is being made on whether or not to do a study. Making n_1, n_2, and/or the difference $P_2 - P_1$ larger will increase the power of a proposed study; but if these numbers were exaggerated by the researcher to give an optimistic result, then resources may be wasted for a study that, in reality, had little chance for success.

Questions:
7. What are α- and β-errors and how do they relate to the performance of the study?
8. If n_1 is the number of cases and n_2 is the number of controls, what are the advantages of increasing these numbers? What are the disadvantages of doing this?
9. How does the expected difference between the occurrence of outcomes among the cases and controls relate to the expected chance of the study to find a statistically significant difference?

Simple Analysis of Case-Control Studies

Dr. M. has completed the study with 400 uninfected (HIV$^-$) controls and 400 infected (HIV$^+$) cases. He obtained the following results: 20/400 cases were diabetics compared with 40/400 controls. From Chapter 8, you should remember how to calculate and interpret an odds ratio from Table 11-1.

To review, the odds ratio is a multiplicate measure of association between the row exposure in Table 11-1 and being a case (rather than a control). In certain settings, the odds ratio closely approximates a multiplicative measure of relative risk (Fleiss, 1981). For example, an odds ratio of 2.0 would mean a diabetic was twice as likely to be HIV infected, while an odds ratio of 0.30 would mean a diabetic was 30% as likely to be infected. From the table, $[a \cdot d/b \cdot c]$ is the point estimate for the odds ratio for a 2×2 table. Now, $\log [a \cdot d/b \cdot c] \pm 1.96 \sqrt{1/a + 1/b + 1/c + 1/d}$ is a 95% confidence interval for the logarithm (base e) of

Table 11-1. Calculation of an odds ratio

	HIV+ Cases	HIV– Controls
Diabetic	$a = 20$	$b = 40$
Nondiabetic	$c = 380$	$d = 360$

the odds ratios, and exponentiating the lower and upper limits of the confidence intervals for the logarithm of the odds ratio obtains lower and upper confidence limits for the odds ratio.

Question:

10. Calculate the odds ratio between HIV-1 infection and diabetes in Table 11-1 with confidence intervals and test this association statistically. Interpret your results.

Confounding

Dr. M. is convinced that this study shows diabetics who inject insulin to be less likely to have HIV infection and that HIV infection can be prevented by periodic injection of insulin into drug users. But other medical implications that would result from insulin injections in nondiabetics make this approach problematic. Furthermore, as described in Chapters 8 and 9, this association could arise from confounding rather than insulin injection's being causally associated with reduced HIV infection. Diabetics could be different from nondiabetics in many ways (other than the use of insulin), which could confound these results. It could be that these other differences, not insulin injection, caused the lower levels of HIV infection in diabetics. Potential confounding factors are that diabetics tend to be (1) older, (2) heavier, and (3) more likely women than nondiabetics. Another potential confounder is that (4) legally diabetics have strong access to the medical care system for needles for the injection of insulin and, therefore, may have less need to rely on shared needles; that is, diabetics can use the clean needles given to them for insulin to inject illicit drugs and thus do not need to seek blood-contaminated needles elsewhere. If any of the factors 1–4 above is itself related to HIV infection, that could create an artificial (confounded) association between self-injected insulin and HIV infection. This association is illustrated in Figure 11-2, for example, with access to clean needles.

It is the easy access to clean needles (hence, less sharing of needles) that is directly associated with reduced HIV infection in this figure. While injected insulin is not causally associated with reduced HIV infection, insulin users have strong access to clean needles, which reduces transmission through shared residual blood.

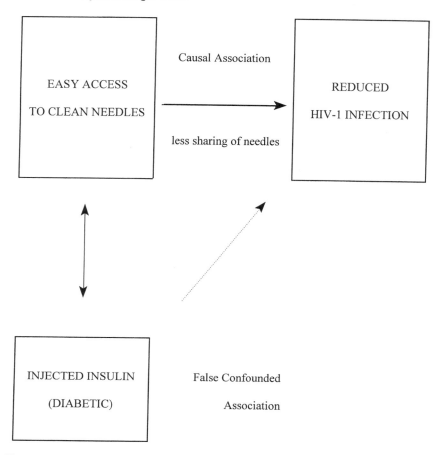

Figure 11-2. Confounded association between self-injected insulin and HIV infection. HIV-1, human immunodeficiency virus type 1.

Question:

11. What are the health policy implications if, in fact, the lower rates of HIV infection among diabetic drug users were due to access to clean needles rather than external insulin?

Statistical and Multivariate Analyses of Confounding

It is possible to investigate and adjust for artificial associations created by confounding through simultaneous comparison of cases and controls based on two or more variables. Details of the many possible statistical methods for this have been given elsewhere (Fleiss, 1981; Thompson, 1994). The simplest form of

Table 11-2. Calculation of odds ratios after stratification by a confounder

	Share Needles ≥ 1 Time/Week		Share Needles < 1 Time/Week	
	HIV+ Case	HIV– Control	HIV+ Case	HIV– Control
Diabetic	12	4	8	36
Nondiabetic	330	110	50	250
	Odds ratio = 1.00		Odds ratio = 1.11	

this approach, used when an exposure covariate (i.e., exposure to insulin) and another categorical (potentially confounding) covariate are involved, is stratified analysis. Separate analyses of the relation between the primary (exposure) covariate of interest and the case-control outcome are performed for data segregated into different levels of the secondary covariate that may be a confounder. For example, let the primary exposure variable be diabetes and the secondary variable be ''share needles at least once per week.'' Consider the following analysis of diabetes vs. case-control status that is stratified by sharing needles.

Within the stratified Table 11-2, we can see that a very different relation exists between diabetes and HIV case-control status than exists in the overall unstratified table. In Table 11-2A, the odds ratio is 1.00, and in B, the odds ratio is 1.11. We can check that the numbers in the stratified tables add up to those of the overall table presented earlier (i.e., 20 total HIV$^+$ diabetics, etc.). Quite simply, the following has happened. Diabetics are not likely to share frequently; only 16/60 (26.7%) did so compared with 440/640 (63.8%) of nondiabetics. However, sharing needles <1/week was protective against HIV-1 disease, as Table 11-3 shows (odds ratio = 0.068, 95% confidence interval 0.048–0.096).

Thus, diabetics who had access to clean needles from the medical community tended not to share needles and, because of this, tended not to become infected with HIV. However, once we separated the individuals into those who did and did not share needles ≥1 time/week, thus removing this confounding, the protective effect of diabetes vanished. Within each stratified table, there was no relation between HIV status and diabetes (i.e., insulin injection).

Table 11-3. Identification of association between a confounding variable and outcome

	HIV+ Case	HIV– Control
Share needles < 1/week	58	286
Share needles ≥ 1/week	342	114
	Odds ratio = 0.068	

Table 11-4. Association between heart disease and marijuana use stratified by smoking tobacco

		Not Smoking Tobacco		Smoking Tobacco	
		Heart Disease		Heart Disease	
		Cases	Controls	Cases	Controls
Use Marijuana	Yes	10	25	70	20
	No	90	220	130	35

Question:

12. An analysis of the relationship between marijuana consumption and heart disease stratified by tobacco smoking is shown in Table 11-4.
    a. Calculate the odds ratios and 95% confidence intervals for the odds ratios in each of the stratified tables.
    b. Pool the numbers in the stratified tables together to create an unstratified table. Calculate the odds ratios and 95% confidence intervals.
    c. Was stratification needed to remove confounding from marijuana users being more likely to smoke tobacco?

Often, there is more than one potential confounder and/or the confounders are continuous (i.e., age) and cannot be categorized. In this setting, stratification is not feasible. Instead, as shown in Chapter 9, multivariate logistic regression models are fit to simultaneously study the effects of multiple potential confounders and to derive better prediction equations (Fleiss, 1981; Thompson, 1994). To simultaneously examine the effect of diabetes, age, gender, and sharing needles ≥ 1 time/week on the probability to be a case, the following model is fit:

$$\log \left[\frac{y}{1-y} \right] = \alpha + \beta_1 x_1 + \beta_2 x_2 + \beta_3 x_3 + \beta_4 x_4$$

where the logarithm taken is the natural (base e) logarithm, y is the probability for an individual from the study population to have HIV infection, x_1 is whether that individual has diabetes ($1 =$ yes, $0 =$ no), x_2 is the person's age in years, x_3 is the person's gender ($1 =$ female, $0 =$ male), and x_4 is the person's sharing needles <1 time/week status ($1 =$ yes, $0 =$ no). The term α is a constant that has no interpretation here, while β_1, β_2, β_3, and β_4, respectively, are constants related to the impact of the covariates x_1, x_2, x_3, x_4, respectively, on the probability of being infected with HIV. By exponentiating β_i, (i.e., $e^{[\beta_i]}$), we obtain the impact on the odds ratio of being infected with HIV from increasing the covariate x_i by one unit.

Table 11-5. Associations between multiple variables and HIV-1[a] seropositivity in a multivariate logistic regression

	Coefficient		
Variable	Estimate[b]	Standard Error	Z Score[c]
Diabetic	0.00	0.25	0.00(1.00)[d]
Age (years)	−0.09	0.04	−2.25(0.027)
Female (gender)	0.31	0.21	1.48(0.14)
Share <1 time/week	−2.03	0.32	−6.34(<0.0001)

[a]HIV, human immunodeficiency virus type 1.

[b]For the effect of the variable on probability to be HIV-seropositive as explained in the text.

[c]The Z score is the ratio of the coefficient estimate to its standard error.

[d]Numbers in parentheses, p values.

For example, fitting this model to the hypothetical case-control study of Dr. M. obtained the point estimates and standard errors shown in Table 11-5.

Thus, after adjustment was made for age, gender, and needle sharing, the multiplicative impact of being a diabetic on the odds ratio for HIV infection was $\exp(0.00) = 1$, or no impact. However, after adjustment was made for diabetes, gender, and needle sharing, the multiplicative impact of being 1 year older on the odds ratio of HIV infection was $\exp(-0.09) = 0.91$. That is, everything else being equal, older drug users were less likely to be infected with HIV. To obtain the impact of being x years older, one can exponentiate this coefficient, 0.91, to the xth. Thus, everything else being equal, an individual who is 10 years older has an odds ratio of $0.39 = (0.91)^{10}$ of being HIV-infected compared with the younger individual.

Confidence limits on the odds ratio are obtained by first constructing confidence limits on the coefficients and then exponentiating those limits. For example:

$$0.07 = \exp^{(-2.03 - 1.96 \times 0.32)} < OR_{Share < 1 \text{ time/week}} < \exp^{(>2.03 + 1.96 \times 0.32)} = 0.25$$

This is a 95% confidence limit for the multiplicative effect of sharing <1 time/week on the odds for being HIV$^+$, everything else being equal. More details on multivariate logistic regression are described elsewhere (Fleiss, 1981).

The coefficients and standard errors shown in Table 11-5 are standard output from most logistic regression analysis procedures available in commercial statistical packages. While the reader should seek further statistical training (or advice from statisticians), he or she will need to become familiar with this type of multivariate analysis to conduct and judge epidemiologic research.

Questions:

13. Calculate the estimated multivariate adjusted impact on odds ratios for HIV-1 infection from (a) being female and from (b) being 5 years older. Calculate the 95% confidence interval for the adjusted impacts of these factors (a) and (b) on the true odds ratio.
14. On the basis of results from this study, what individuals should be tar-geted the most for intervention programs against HIV infection ?
15. Does this study prove that diabetes is not related to HIV after adjusting for other factors? If not, what additional information would you like to see [hint: confidence interval]?

It should be noted that Nelson et al. (1991) did, in fact, find that diabetic drug users had lower rates of HIV infection than did other drug users and concluded that availability of clean needles was the major reason for this.

Prospective Studies and Observational Studies of Intervention

As was described previously, very early in the HIV epidemic, an overwhelming amount of biologic, case investigation, and case-control study evidence implicated shared needles as a major route of HIV transmission (Hoover, 1996; Merrigan and Balognesi, 1993; Normand et al., 1995). The next step in resolving this major health problem is using this information to develop strategies for reducing the spread of HIV among intravenous drug users. While it is not difficult to think of intervention mechanisms to break the shared needle route of transmission, the cost-effectiveness of such ideas must be tested using prospective (and observational) studies.

Two potential approaches to reduce needle-borne transmission of HIV among drug users are the following:

Approach A. Cause people to stop using intravenous drugs. This would require behavior modification programs that cause people to quit using drugs with needles or prevent them from initiating drug use by needles.
Approach B. Help people to use clean needles (with no contamination from previous users) when they inject. This requires methods to facilitate the availability of clean needles so that individuals who inject drugs can do so without transmitting HIV.

From a historical standpoint, it should be noted that behavioral programs to curb drug use have been attempted over the past 30 years (Latkin et al., 1993; Normand et al., 1995) without much success. In particular, individuals addicted to drugs have such a strong dependency that even the fear of contracting a fatal disease will not alter behavior. Thus, approach A may be difficult.

Facilitating the availability of clean needles (approach B) can be accomplished either by (1) providing chemicals that will kill HIV on residual blood inside previously used needles and syringes or (2) providing fresh, unused needles. It was shown in laboratory studies that chlorine bleach killed HIV virus in residual blood left in previously used needles. However, programs to provide and educate injection drug users to use bleach to clean needles have had mixed results (Vlahov et al., 1994). Problems have included nonuse and misuse of bleach due to inconvenience and the fact that even simple steps may be difficult to take by someone under the influence of drugs. A more promising approach has been the concept of needle exchange. Centers are set up where drug users can return old, used needles. For each used needle they bring in, a fresh unused needle is given back. Because needles are cheap, such programs are inexpensive and easy to operate. However, as with any health services program, potential deleterious side effects from providing exchange needles must be considered. In particular, one cannot ignore the possibility that making unused needles readily available could cause more harm than good by facilitating and encouraging the use of illicit drugs.

Several needle exchange programs have been conducted in the United States and in Europe. A committee of the Institute of Medicine recently concluded from data on these programs that exchanging needles can reduce HIV transmission without increasing drug use (Normand et al., 1995). We now present the results of an illustrative clinical trial (clinical trials are covered in Chapter 9) on the effectiveness of a needle exchange program.

Clinical Trials

Dr. S. studied whether making clean needles available (by exchange) for clients who returned used needles would (1) reduce the incidence of HIV infection and/ or (2) reduce the cessation of drug use. The requirement to return a used needle to get a clean needle ensures that a dirty needle is returned for each clean needle provided. Thus new needles are not being added to the supply. She enrolled 400 high-risk injection drug users who were not infected with HIV and who attended the same outreach drug rehabilitation clinic. Two hundred of these users were randomly assigned to a group that was provided clean needles in exchange for used needles. The other 200 did not have this option, but all 400 continued to be monitored and given the drug cessation education provided by the clinic.

Two outcome events were evaluated in this study: (1) seroconversion to HIV (for which tests were done regularly) was compared between study groups to see if exchange needles would reduce this and (2) cessation of drug use (based on negative urine tests) was evaluated to see if making needles available would hinder this. The study began in January 1990 and ended in December 1995. Subjects were recruited throughout the 6-year period. A substantial number of

HIV seroconversions ($n = 50$) occurred during this study. Not all individuals in the study could be followed for the same length of time; an individual recruited in January 1990 could be followed for 6 years to see if HIV infection occurred, while one recruited in January 1995 could be followed only for 1 year. Clearly, the former person has more time and chance to become infected.

When study subjects are followed for different lengths of time, statistical comparisons that adjust for this must be used (Cox and Oakes, 1984). One commonly used longitudinal approach is proportional hazards models. The full statistical details of these methods are beyond the scope of this chapter but are covered in statistical textbooks (Cox and Oakes, 1984). We focus on explaining what the results of proportional hazards models mean and how these models are used.

The "hazard" of HIV seroconversion is a mathematic quantification of the rate of HIV infection. A higher hazard means a higher rate of infection. Often, the ratios of hazards are used to compare risks under a proportional hazards assumption. If the ratio of person B's hazard to person A's hazard is 2.0, this means that over a short period of time person B is twice as likely to become infected as person A.

A proportional hazards assumption means that the effect of a characteristic on the risk of an outcome is to multiply the hazard for that outcome by a specific amount. For example, if male gender exerts a proportional effect on the hazards of 2.0, then, everything else being equal, a man has twice the hazard of an identical female; that is, a 39-year-old man who uses a needle exchange program has twice the hazard to contract HIV as a 39-year-old woman who uses a needle exchange program. Similarly, a 23-year-old man who does not use a needle exchange program has twice the hazard as a 23-year-old woman who does not use the program. Statistical methods exist to estimate the logarithm (base e) of a variable's effect on the hazard ratio when the assumption of a proportional hazards model is true. The standard error of these estimates also can be obtained.

Dr. S. fit the following proportional hazards model:

$$\log \begin{bmatrix} Hazard \\ HIV \\ Infection \end{bmatrix} = \alpha + \beta_1 x_1 + \beta_2 x_2 + \beta_3 x_3$$

where x_1 indicates whether the person was randomized to the exchange program ($0 = $ no, $1 = $ yes); x_2 is the person's gender ($0 = $ male, $1 = $ female); x_3 is the person's age; α is a constant that has no direct interpretation; and β_1, β_2, and β_3 are numeric coefficients of the logarithm of the respective covariates (exchange program, gender, and age) effect on the hazard of HIV infection. The estimates in Table 11-6 were obtained from statistical analysis of Dr. S.'s data.

The Z score is the ratio of the coefficient estimate to the standard error. Since

Table 11-6. Associations of variables with hazard of HIV seroconversion in a multivariate proportional hazards model

	Coefficient		
Variable	Estimate[a]	Standard Error	Z score
Needle exchange group	−2.01	0.35	−5.74 (<0.0001)[b]
Female gender	0.69	0.24	2.87 (0.005)
Age (per year)	0.00	0.04	0.00 (1.00)

[a] For the logarithm of the variable effect on the hazard ratio of HIV infection.

[b] Numbers in parentheses, p values.

exponentiation is the inverse function of taking logarithms, exponentiation of the coefficients (for logarithm of effects) gives the multiplicative effect of the covariate on the hazard ratio for the outcome (HIV seroconversion). Thus, everything else (age and gender) being equal, a person in the needle exchange group was less likely to become infected with HIV. During a short time period, this person has 0.13 ($e^{[−2.01]}$) times the hazard of seroconverting to HIV as one not in the exchange group. This means that, everything else being equal, over a short time interval, an uninfected person in the exchange program was 0.13 times as likely to become infected with HIV as one not in the exchange program. However, a woman was more likely than a man to become infected with HIV (relative hazard $1.99 = e^{[0.69]}$), everything else being equal. Age was not statistically important in this study, the relative hazard being $1.00 = e^{[0.00]}$, meaning that seroconversion rates were the same for all ages.

As with the odds ratio in logistic regression, a 95% confidence interval for the true effect of the covariate on the hazard ratio can be obtained by exponentiating the lower and upper limits of the 95% confidence interval for the coefficient. Thus:

$$\exp^{(0.00 - 1.96 \times 0.04)} < RH_{year} < \exp^{(0.00 + 1.96 \times 0.04)}$$

or $0.925 < RH_{year} < 1.08$, where RH_{year} represents the impact of a 1-year increase in age on the hazard of HIV seroconversion.

To determine the effect of an increase in age by x years on the hazard of HIV seroconversion, we would exponentiate the hazards of a 1-year change to the x power. Thus, the 95% confidence interval for the effect of an increase in 10 years of age on the hazard is $0.46 - 2.16$; $0.45 = (0.925)^{10}$, $2.16 = (1.08)^{10}$.

Based on this multivariate analysis, the needle exchange program has been beneficial toward reducing HIV infection in this group with statistical certainty ($p < 0.0001$). Furthermore, the magnitude of the effect has been tremendous, cutting the hazard of transmission by almost 90%. However, further analysis is needed to quantify the cost benefits of this program. In particular, we would need to estimate the following:

- The number of HIV infections prevented by the availability of needles in the exchange group (The relative hazard does not directly give this, but other methods [Cox and Oakes, 1984] could be used to estimate it.)
- The costs per person-year of the exchange program (If the program is too expensive, it will not be feasible.)
- The generalizability of this study to injection needle drug users other than those in the particular clinic population used for this study (It is possible that the particular group studied would utilize clean exchange needles to a greater [or lesser] degree than would other injection drug users.)

While all of these are very important for evaluating the potential benefits of a needle exchange intervention, no standardized approach exists for answering the questions posed in the estimates above using data from a single prospective study. Rather, as will be described in Chapter 12, several studies in different settings will need to be completed and compared.

Another issue, noted earlier, that needs to be explored is whether the needle exchange program was associated with reduced likelihood to quit drugs. Remember, one possibility is that the supply of clean needles from an exchange program will remove incentives to quit using drugs. In questions 16–18, the reader is asked to study this issue based on a proportional hazards analysis of the cessation of drug use among the 400 individuals in Dr. S.'s study. Remember, the outcome of this analysis, cessation of drug use, is a desirable event (Table 11-7).

Questions:
16. Does this analysis suggest that increasing the availability of clean needles through an exchange program will reduce the likelihood to quit drugs?
17. Give a point estimate and 95% confidence limits for the relative hazard of females (vs. males) to quit drugs, age and exchange group status being equal.

Table 11-7. Associations of variables with cessation of drug use in a multivariate proportional hazards model

| Variable | Coefficient | | | |
	Estimate[a]	Standard Error	Z Score	p Value
Needle exchange group (1 = yes, 0 = no)	0.15	0.30	0.50	0.62
Female gender (1 = yes, 0 = no)	−0.33	0.19	−1.73	0.08
Age (per year)	−0.07	0.03	−2.33	0.02

[a]For the variable effect on the logarithm of the hazard ratio for cessation of drug use.

18. What individuals does this analysis suggest will be the most receptive to a program for drug use cessation? (Remember, these study participants were enrolled in a drug use cessation program.)
19. What are the health policy implications for the results presented in Tables 11-6 and 11-7 and the analysis just described?

Summary

This chapter has sought to illustrate the analytic aspects for the application of epidemiologic research of health services interest and testing solutions. We have illustrated many of the analytic methods described in the previous chapters, particularly Chapters 6–9. We began with case studies that drew the problem to the attention of the scientific community and ended with a clinical trial for testing a solution. The ultimate decision on whether to implement this solution (a needle exchange program) would depend on principles described in Chapter 4 and on the magnitude of the health problem (AIDS in drug users), as determined by methods described in Chapters 5 and 10. However, one clinical trial will not be sufficient to determine whether a needle exchange program will work. Several clinical trials will need to be conducted and compared. The methods to do this are the focus of the final chapter of this book.

Question:
20. What are the analytic tools we described for the following:
    a. case investigations
    b. deciding whether research will be cost-effective
    c. case-control studies
    d. treatment of confounding in case-control studies
    e. clinical trials

Answers to Questions

1. The purpose of case investigations is to identify determinants of a current or potential problem with medical significance as we learn from individual cases/patients. All attributes related to cause, identification, and prevention should be described.
2. The key hypothesis of the report is that the causal agent of AIDS may be spread by needles shared among drug users.
3. The analytic methods used in this investigation are the description, identification, and presentation of characteristics that make these cases unique and shed light on their etiology.
4. Additional information that should have been reported is: (i) the serologic

results for HIV testing, if such tests were available at the time, to support the hypothesized chain of transmission; (ii) the AIDS status of Mrs. S.'s husband and his friends, to support the hypothesized initial source; and (iii) the present history of sexually transmitted diseases for Miss R. or verification that none existed, to support the contention that AIDS was not acquired sexually.

5. Based on this case report, additional approaches to ascertain medical significance would be to learn about the number of injection drug users, the number who share needles, and the role of shared needles in the spread of HIV/AIDS and to conduct case-control studies of the importance of shared needles.

6. Population studies both are more expensive and take longer to finish than do case-control and cross-sectional studies. Thus, case-control and cross-sectional studies are more cost-effective as methods for rapid acquisition of information.

7. An α-error is rejecting the null hypothesis (i.e., no difference of disease between the two groups) when it is true. A β-error is failing to reject the null hypothesis when it is false (i.e., there really is a difference in rate of disease between two groups). The smaller the chances for making α- and β-errors, the better a study is.

8. Increasing n_1 and n_2 increases the costs of a study (a disadvantage) but lowers the α- and β-errors of that study (an advantage).

9. Everything else being equal (i.e., n_1 controls, n_2 cases, and a given α-error), the greater this difference is, the smaller the β-error is and, thus, the larger $(1 - \beta)$, or power (the expected chance to find a difference), is.

10. The calculations are as follow:

$$\text{OR} = \frac{a \cdot d}{b \cdot c} = \frac{20 \cdot 360}{40 \cdot 380} = 0.47$$

$$95\% \text{ CI} = \exp\left[\ln\left[\frac{a\,d}{c\,d} \right] \pm 1.96 \sqrt{\frac{1}{a} + \frac{1}{b} + \frac{1}{c} + \frac{1}{d}} \right]$$

$$= \exp\left[-0.75 \pm 0.56\right]$$

$$= (0.27, 0.83)$$

A diabetic drug user is estimated to have 47% percent the chance that a nondiabetic drug user has to be infected with HIV infection. With 95% certainty, the range of this chance is 27–83%.

11. This has tremendous policy importance. Providing external insulin to nondiabetic drug users would be both costly and productive of medical side effects. This would be a mistake if the focus of the prevention program should be providing clean needles to at-risk drug users.

12. The odds ratios, unstratified table, and conclusion are as follows:

    a. Odds ratios for marijuana use and heart disease:
    Nontobacco smokers:

    $$OR = 0.98$$
    $$95\% \text{ CI } 0.45\text{--}2.11$$

    Tobacco smokers:·

    $$OR = 0.94$$
    $$95\% \text{ CI } 0.51\text{--}1.75$$

    b. Combined odds ratios:

    | | | Heart Disease | |
		Cases	Controls
Marijuana Use	Yes	80	45
	No	220	255

    OR (95% CI)
    2.06 (1.38–3.07)

    c. In the preceding combined table, the lower limit for the 95% confidence interval between marijuana use and heart disease is greater than 1, suggesting that marijuana use is a risk factor for heart disease. However, in the stratified tables, the odds ratios between marijuana use and heart disease are very close to 1. What has happened is that smoking tobacco is related to both heart disease and marijuana use, making marijuana use associated with heart disease by confounding.

13. The calculated odds ratios are as follows:

    a. Being female:

    $$1.36 = \exp(0.31)$$
    $$95\% \text{ CI } 0.90 = \exp(0.31 - 1.96 \, [0.21])$$
    $$2.06 = \exp(0.31 + 1.96 \, [0.21])$$

    b. Being 5 years older:

    $$0.64 = [\exp(-0.09)]^5$$
    $$95\% \text{ CI } 0.43 = [\exp(-0.09 - 1.96[0.04])]^5$$
    $$0.94 = [\exp(-0.09 + 1.96[0.04])]^5$$

14. Those who share needles ≥ 1 time per week. The odds ratio for HIV infection for those who share <1 time per week is 0.13, with a 95% confidence interval of 0.07–0.25. This means that most infections occur in those sharing ≥ 1 time per week. If causality can be shown, then reduction of needle sharing could reduce substantially HIV-1 infection.

15. The 95% confidence interval for the adjusted effect of diabetes on the odds of HIV infection is 0.61–1.63. Therefore, it is possible that diabetes could still have a substantial effect. If this study was repeated using a larger number of cases and controls, the confidence intervals would be narrower, providing a more accurate picture of the adjusted effect of diabetes on risk of HIV infection.

16. No, the estimated effect of being in the needle exchange group on cessation of drug use was slightly positive, $\exp (0.15) = 1.16$, meaning that individuals in the needle exchange program were slightly more likely to quit drug use than others. However, the lower 95% confidence limits for this effect were $\exp (0.15 – 1.96 \cdot 0.30) = 0.65$, meaning that participants in needle exchange programs still could be slightly less likely to quit drug usage.

17. Point estimate:

$$\exp(-0.33) = 0.72, \text{ 95% confidence limit}$$
$$[\exp(-0.33 – 1.96 \cdot 0.19), \exp(-0.33 + 1.96 \cdot 0.19)] = (0.50 \text{ to } 1.04)$$

18. The coefficient estimate for age was negative, and the p value (0.02) was significant (less than 0.05). This means that older drug users had lower hazard rates for quitting drugs than younger users. Thus, younger users were more likely to quit drugs and *may be* benefitting more from the drug cessation program. Females also had lower hazards ($p = 0.08$) for quitting drugs, suggesting that men were more likely to quit.

19. This suggests that a needle exchange program will reduce HIV-1 infection without increasing drug use. Other factors that must be considered before implementing such a program include the following:
    a. cost-effectiveness
    b. generalizability to other populations
    c. alternate methods
    d. other priorities for health services

20. The analytic tools described are as follows:
    a. descriptive methods
    b. power sample size calculations
    c. 2×2 tables, odds ratios, confidence intervals
    d. stratified analysis, multivariate logistic regression
    e. proportional hazards models, hazard rates, confidence intervals

Acknowledgment

The author appreciates support from the National Institute of Drug Abuse, grants 04334 and 10184, for this research.

References

Benenson, A. S. 1995. *Control of Communicable Diseases in Man,* 32nd ed. Washington, D.C.: American Public Health Association.

Cox, D. R., and D. Oakes. 1984. *Analysis of Survival Data.* London: Chapman and Hall.

Fleiss, J. L. 1981. *Statistical Methods for Rates and Proportions.* New York: John Wiley & Sons.

Hoover, D. R., M. C. Doherty, D. Vlahov, et al. 1996. Incidence and risk factors for HIV-1 infection: a summary of what is known and the psychiatric relevance. *Int. Rev. Psychiatry,* 8:137–148.

Latkin, C. A., D. Vlahov, and J. Anthony. 1993. Socially desirable responding and self-reported HIV infection risk behaviors among intravenous drug users. *Br. J. Addiction,* 88:517–526.

Merrigan, T. C., and D. Balognesi, eds. 1993. *Textbook of AIDS Medicine.* Baltimore: William & Wilkins.

Nelson, K. E., D. Vlahov, S. Cohn, et al. 1991. Human immunodeficiency virus infection in diabetic intravenous drug users. *JAMA,* 266:2259–2261.

Normand, J., D. Vlahov, and L. E. Moses, eds. 1995. *Preventing HIV Transmission— The Role of Sterile Needles and Bleach.* Washington, D.C.: National Academy Press.

Shilts, R. 1987. *And the Band Played On.* New York: Penguin Books.

Shuster, J. J. 1990. *Handbook of Sample Size Guidelines for Clinical Trials.* Boca Raton, FL: CRC Press.

Thompson, W. D. 1994. Statistical analysis of case-control studies. *Epidemiol. Rev.,* 16:33–50.

Vlahov, D. J., J. Astemborski, L. Solomon, et al. 1994. Field effectiveness of needle exchange among injection drug users. *J. Acquir. Immune. Defic. Syndr.,* 9:743–746.

Chapter 12

Meta-analysis in Health Services Research

Steven N. Goodman

Meta-analysis is possibly the most important policy-related research method that has developed in the past two decades. The term "meta-analysis" appeared in 1976 in the psychology literature; George Glass defined it as "the statistical analysis of a large collection of results from individual studies for the purpose of integrating the findings" (Glass, 1976). However, even though the name and some of the formal methodology are fairly new, particularly in the biomedical field, such analysis has been practiced in some form in a variety of settings for many years. The practice of bringing together all of the relevant research in an area to inform a debate about a policy hardly started with the coining of the term "meta-analysis." However, the development of meta-analysis as a formal method has introduced a certain degree of rigor, consistency, and, most important, a new awareness among health researchers of the importance of combined analysis of research studies addressing similar topics.

Before discussing the techniques of meta-analysis, we must first understand what it is. A good meta-analysis has two parts: a qualitative component and a quantitative one. The qualitative component can be seen as a form of descriptive epidemiology, with individual studies serving as the research subjects. The existing research in an area is first found and described, and its characteristics are analyzed. The results of this procedure are formally presented. In the quantitative component, studies that focus on similar enough subjects, interventions, and outcomes and have similar enough designs are combined to produce a pooled estimate of effect, which is usually more precise than could be provided by any of the individual studies.

The simple and somewhat naive view of the purpose of meta-analysis is that it is a way to obtain a "definitive" verdict on the efficacy of an intervention by combining all of the research in an area, thereby creating a pseudoexperiment of very large sample size that will have a precision adequate to discern differences that individual studies might miss. Another closely related view is that it is useful to "resolve differences" between apparently conflicting studies. Neither perspective is completely correct, but these views of meta-analysis have fueled controversy and criticism of the technique since both put the method in direct competition with the studies on which it is based. To the extent that individual studies are seen just as potential contributors to a meta-analysis, without much intrinsic value, it is understandable that researchers who conduct such studies might resent seeing their years of work reduced to a single "effect size" for entry in a rapidly done "definitive" analysis by someone unknown in their field.

A more seasoned view of the purpose of meta-analyses is expressed by one of the alternate terms that has been widely used to describe them: "systematic overviews." A meta-analysis is a comprehensive description, including strengths and weaknesses, of the body of evidence in a particular field. Sometimes its most valuable contribution is to demonstrate that the state of the research is such that no policy can be said to have adequate scientific justification. Similarly, the outcome of some meta-analyses is to point the way toward new avenues of research or ways to improve on the research that has been done. To the extent that this evidence can be quantitatively combined, the meta-analysis has correspondingly greater value, but ultimately it is only as useful as the qualitative picture of the evidence that it can provide, which depends on the sophistication of the statistical/scientific judgments that go into deciding if and when research can be combined.

A recent working group in environmental epidemiology (Blair et al., 1995) outlined a range of functions for meta-analysis, which is modified here for health services research:

- identify heterogeneity in effects among multiple studies and, where appropriate, provide summary statistics that portray the relationship between a health service and consequent health effects
- increase statistical power to detect an effect over that of individual studies, which are limited by the rarity of an outcome or the small number of subjects
- develop, refine, and test hypotheses
- provide the basis for identifying beneficial or harmful health interventions, or identify critical components of an intervention that account for most of its effect
- reduce the subjectivity of study comparisons by using systematic and explicit comparison procedures
- identify data gaps in the knowledge base and suggest directions for future research

Before we take a more detailed look at this methodology, it must be stressed that often the most valuable, if not the only, product of a meta-analysis is the qualitative component. To provide an informed, comprehensive, and structured portrait of the research literature is difficult, and it can be an extremely valuable contribution by itself. If the existing studies are not combinable, that is as far as one can go. In the rush to produce an analysis, however, the qualitative component is sometimes either ignored or given cursory attention.

The most active area of meta-analysis in medicine is with randomized clinical trials. The reason for this is clear: because of the randomization process, these trials are generally considered to provide unbiased, internally valid results. That is, even if the populations studied in two randomized clinical trials are different, the measure of effect used in each should be unbiased, and, as long as it is not thought to be appreciably different in the two populations, the two estimates can be combined to give a more precise estimate. In observational studies, the application of meta-analysis is more problematic because we can never be sure that the two populations being compared have equal risk profiles. As a result, there has been comparatively little meta-analysis of health services studies compared with the evaluation of medical interventions that have been tested in a randomized fashion.

The description of the basics of meta-analysis below is structured around a study of the possible benefits (or harms) of electronic fetal monitoring (Thacker et al., 1995). We then briefly look at another published meta-analysis, of the utility of stroke units in reducing mortality (Langhorne et al., 1993).

Electronic fetal monitoring consists of the placement of electrodes on the scalp of an unborn child while the child is still in the uterus, which allows a continuous electronic monitoring of the fetal heart rate through the course of labor. The rationale for this procedure is that it allows a physician to react promptly to any indication of fetal distress. The traditional alternative to electronic fetal monitoring is intermittent auscultation, that is, listening to the fetal heartbeat every 15–30 min through a special stethoscope placed on the pregnant woman's abdomen.

While electronic fetal monitoring is not a typical health services intervention, it is actually quite similar. It is not a therapy itself but rather serves a screening function, acting as a potential trigger for a range of medical interventions (e.g., hospital monitoring, cesarean deliveries) that differ depending on the setting and are not determined by the monitoring. Assessing this procedure is essentially a programmatic evaluation of the clinical outcomes from the medical and institutional responses to this means of following labor.

The following general outline for the conduct and assessment of a meta-analysis will serve as the framework for examining this example:

1. Composition of the research team
2. Framing the question
3. Searching the literature

4. Study eligibility
5. Qualitative data abstraction and presentation
6. Qualitative meta-analysis
7. Quality scoring
8. Quantitative data abstraction
9. Quantitative meta-analysis
10. Limitations, conclusions, and implications

Composition of the Research Team

One of the areas that rarely receives mention in descriptions of meta-analytic methods is the makeup of the team that will conduct the meta-analysis. It is critical that this team have individuals with at least two forms of expertise: content expertise, preferably not derived just from reading the studies to be meta-analyzed, and methodologic expertise, both in the methods to assess study quality and in the implementation and interpretation of the statistical methods to combine study results. It cannot be emphasized too strongly how important it is to have individuals who can make nuanced and informed judgments in each of these domains. The following judgments come at every stage of a meta-analysis: how the question can be framed, how to find the relevant literature, deciding which studies to include, deciding which subsidiary questions and study subsets should be explored, determining the most important aspects of study quality, assessing whether the sometimes subtle differences between studies prevent them from being combined, and presenting and interpreting the statistical summaries.

Framing the Question

One of the critical aspects of a meta-analysis is a proper framing of the question to be asked. In particular, it must be a question that could reasonably be addressed using meta-analytic methodology. This generally means that, at least, there should be a clearly definable intervention and outcome, whose relation has been addressed in empirical studies. An example is whether antibiotic prophylaxis before abdominal surgery reduces postsurgical morbidity and mortality. Even as I present that, however, a reader may begin to ask questions: What kind of prophylaxis? What kind of surgery? What kinds of morbidity? Mortality within what time frame and due to what cause? How these questions are answered is a matter of scientific judgment and will be another focus of our discussion.

Questions that are not appropriate for meta-analysis are those that address broad areas of mechanism, process, or the efficacy of a multitude of interventions with many different kinds of outcome. In medicine, this type of question could be one of the following: What is the mechanism linking high blood cholesterol to heart attacks? Does improved emergency medical technician training benefit the community? We could imagine narrower questions within those domains that might be amenable to meta-analysis, but, as posed, a meta-analysis might not be the best tool to elucidate them.

Framing a question for meta-analysis has two components: (1) establishing the context within current practice that defines the motivation for the meta-analysis and its potential importance and (2) defining the specific intervention (and comparison method, if relevant) and outcomes to be studied.

The authors of the meta-analysis of electronic fetal monitoring do this in the first paragraphs of their introduction:

> Electronic fetal monitoring (EFM) is used in the management of labor and delivery in nearly three of four pregnancies in the United States. In 1988, ACOG [American College of Obstetrics and Gynecology] issued a policy statement that recommended either EFM or intermittent auscultation as alternatives in low-risk pregnancies; however, the United States Preventive Services Task Force and the Canadian Task Force on the Periodic Health Examination reserved EFM for high-risk pregnancies. . . . The apparent contradiction between the widespread use of EFM and expert recommendations to limit routine use indicates that a reassessment of this practice is warranted. (Thacker et al., 1995)

The authors have given us a clear motivation for this meta-analysis: that even though expert opinion appears to be divided, the technology is in widespread use. Clearly, an up-to-date examination of the scientific foundation for this practice is needed. They continue, stating in general terms how they framed their question:

> We compared the efficacy of routine electronic fetal monitoring with that of auscultation through a review of the published randomized controlled clinical trials (RCTs). We examined several measures of morbidity and mortality as well as complications (e.g., operative deliveries). (Thacker et al., 1995)

This passage names the intervention being studied, the type of use (routine, i.e., all cases), the practice it will be compared to (auscultation), the type of evidence that will be used to assess it (published randomized clinical trials), and the range of outcomes examined—mortality, morbidity, and complications. The operational definitions of these terms must be clarified, but this is sufficient to set the stage.

Searching the Literature

Once we define the question, we can start the search for published studies. The literature search for all relevant research on an issue can be quite difficult. The coding of articles in electronic data bases, the terminology used in titles and abstracts, and even the description of research methods within the body of a published paper are highly variable. Thus, multiple search strategies must be used and described adequately in the final report. For all but the simplest searches, a librarian experienced in electronic data base search should help the investigators. These authors said the following:

> Methods: Relevant RCTs were identified by searching MEDLINE (for the period 1966–1994, using multiple terms), contacting experts, and reviewing references in published reports; the completeness of our search was verified though contact with investigators at the Cochrane Collaboration, an international network of investigators that prepares, maintains, and disseminates systematic reviews (i.e., meta-analyses) of studies affecting health care delivery. Unpublished studies were also sought through these sources. (Thacker et al., 1995)

Although this description might have been condensed because of journal space limitations, it is not an adequate description of a search procedure. The criterion that the reader should be able to roughly replicate the process is not fulfilled. We are not told what search terms were used and whether they were used to search titles, key words, or abstracts. Only one data base was studied, calling the completeness of the search into question. In addition, there is no indication that conference proceedings or abstracts were detectable with this process or that searches for other review articles on the topic were conducted. For devices such as the human uterine activity monitor (HUAM), which is made by only one company, it is sometimes of value to ask the manufacturer's representatives if they know of studies. They frequently have access to research that is not submitted for publication. If they refuse to share this, that is a clue that they may be systematically suppressing a body of important information.

The aspects of this description that are strong are the fact that references of cited articles were searched and that the Cochrane Collaboration data base was consulted. Exploration of references of articles found electronically is absolutely essential. Several studies have shown that even optimal electronic search strategies can miss 30–70% of literature that is in MEDLINE (Dickersin et al., 1985, 1990), so supplementation with a hand search of references is mandatory.

The Cochrane Collaboration is described by the authors, and its most comprehensive data base of trials is found in the area of perinatal medicine (Bero and Rennie, 1995). This data base, which started as the Oxford Database of Perinatal Trials in the mid-1980s, is a painstakingly assembled electronic compendium of all randomized trials conducted on perinatal topics, organized by clinical question, and presented in the form of structured meta-analyses. The basis of the data base was a hand search of all journals publishing perinatal research, a worldwide mailing to researchers and practitioners to identify any trials missed in the hand searching, and extensive electronic data base searching; so if we are fortunate enough to be examining a subject covered by the Cochrane data base, it is quite likely that the search will be complete or, at least, will not have missed significant trials on the subject of interest. Although a description of the search is not adequate to replicate it, the reader in this case can have a fair degree of confidence that most, if not all, relevant randomized clinical trials were found.

It is in this phase that the problem of ''publication bias'' may be confronted. Publication bias is the failure of studies that have similar results to be published. The most frequent situation where this is seen is in small studies that show no effectiveness. The fault for the failure to publish is usually in the hands of the researcher, not the editors of journals (Dickersin et al., 1991). Although this can be explored using some quantitative techniques, only direct contact with possible investigators and follow-up of abstracts or proposals can provide proof that it is occurring.

The following statements summarize the main issues in searching the literature:

1. Assistance by medical librarian
2. Use of multiple electronic data bases
3. Clearly described electronic search strategy
4. At least a one- and possibly a two-generation reference search of research and narrative reviews of the topic
5. Nonelectronic sources of data (conference proceedings, abstracts, government reports or studies)
6. Use of the Cochrane Collaboration data base
7. Search for proprietary technology assessment reports in the public domain
8. Search for nonpublished research done by private companies or institutes
9. An attempt to access non-English literature

Study Eligibility

Typically, there are two stages to the search, just as there are in an observational study. A certain number of studies are found by the search strategy, and these are further culled by applying eligibility criteria. This is how the results of this were reported in the paper we are examining:

> We identified 12 RCTs that addressed the efficacy and safety of EFM. . . . The 12 RCTs reviewed in this report addressed eligibility criteria (except the first Melbourne study), described the clinical regimens, provided well-defined end points, used appropriate statistics to measure the main outcomes of interest, and reported the complications of monitoring. (Thacker et al., 1995)

We are not told how many studies were found in the initial search, what specific eligibility criteria were applied, and how many trials were excluded based on which criteria. This is important because it can give a sense of how much and what kind of other work has been done in a field. It might be important to know if there were 35 non-randomized comparative trials in this area. It is implied that only randomized controlled trials were considered, but what we do not know is whether trials that included electronic fetal monitoring but not auscultation were performed, how multiple publications on the same populations were handled, and how random assignment was ascertained, which is frequently not clear in published reports.

Study eligibility should be defined so that the criteria can be applied by any researcher and the same studies admitted and so that it is apparent how variable the selection of studies would be with different criteria. However, even seemingly clear criteria, like randomization, can be so poorly described in a report that the interpretation is ambiguous. This requires that, when possible, at least two persons review articles for eligibility, with a formal procedure for resolving differences.

The following summarizes the main issues in assessing study eligibility:

1. Clearly stated operational criteria
2. Criteria to resolve ambiguities or incompleteness in reporting
3. Two or more assessors, with procedures to resolve disagreement
4. A report of the number of studies assessed and the reasons for disqualification

Qualitative Data Abstraction and Presentation

The goal of this component is to give the reader an objective and comprehensive summary of the literature pertaining to the question at hand. Using again the analogy of an observational study on human subjects, we must first decide what data are needed to describe the population. These descriptive data are typically presented in the first table of a meta-analysis. The electronic fetal monitoring meta-analysis did this in a partially structured way, informally describing the literature in the narrative text and including several design-related details in the table of results. However, these do not present all of the qualitative aspects of the studies in a single format that makes it easy to compare the studies. An example of a fairly complete list of qualitative aspects, presented in a single table, is a 1994 examination of meta-analyses of oral contraceptives and the development of rheumatoid arthritis (Pladevall-Vila et al., 1996). The following study characteristics were reported:

1. Year
2. Site (e.g., outpatient clinic, inpatients, etc.)
3. Country
4. Source and type of cases
5. Source of controls (hospital vs. population)
6. Source of exposure data (e.g., questionnaire vs. medical record)

7. Year of birth of subjects
8. Age at study
9. Confounders that were measured
10. Method of adjustment
11. Outcome criteria
12. Losses to follow-up

Friedenreich (1993) provides a list of issues to consider in the qualitative analysis of epidemiologic studies. The factors that are included should be all those that might affect the quantitative outcome of the study, the interpretation of that outcome, the decision of whether the studies are similar enough to be combined, and the definition of the population to which the results can (or cannot) be generalized. It is rare that this list can be compiled by only one person or before review of the relevant literature. This is where it is absolutely necessary to have someone with good content expertise involved in the investigation.

Like study eligibility, there is potential variability in the data abstraction procedure, so it is sometimes recommended that more than one abstractor be used for the same studies and that the reliability of the abstraction be assessed.

The following summarizes the main data abstraction issues:

1. Compile a list of all elements related to the setting of the study, study design, patient characteristics, and operational definition of critical variables (i.e., quality and completeness of data gathering)
2. Revise the list after reading relevant studies
3. Assess the reliability of data abstraction
4. Present qualitative data in a clearly readable, tabular format, either by individual study or grouped (if the number of studies makes it impractical to present individual data)

Qualitative Meta-analysis

Now we come to the central intellectual component of a meta-analysis—the qualitative part. If the exposition of the study details and analysis of trial quality have been adequate, this section need not be very difficult or lengthy. This part has two functions: (1) to describe any important patterns or differences in design or quality within the research studies and (2) to justify the combining of studies in the quantitative part and to provide the motivation and structure for later sensitivity analysis or analysis of confounders.

The meta-analysis of electronic fetal monitoring does not specifically label it as such but has some components of a qualitative meta-analysis in two sections: the end of the methods section, which outlines the subgroup analyses they plan to perform, and before a "summary outcomes" section, where they look at the "outcomes of individual clinical trials." The following is reported in the sub-group analysis section:

> We performed subgroup analysis for five groups of studies: 1) all RCTs comparing routine EFM with auscultation, 2) studies in which EFM was performed without fetal scalp sampling, 3) studies in which EFM was performed with fetal scalp sampling, 4) studies with low, medium, and high-quality scores, and 5) US and non-US studies. (Thacker et al., 1995)

In this section, the authors have implicitly laid out, before conducting the analysis, what design confounders they anticipate: type of sampling, quality of study, and country in which the study was done. This sets the stage for a qualitative analysis that considers the extent to which these factors might be correlated with each other, which is often the case. That is, were the non-U.S. studies of higher quality, or did all U.S. studies use fetal scalp sampling? This was not done, though some of it can be gleaned from the section on individual study results, which states, albeit nonsystematically, some of the design features of the individual studies. However, the focus in that section was not to justify later combinability or to give a qualitative portrait of the literature.

Ideally, the qualitative aspects of the studies being analyzed should be laid out in a large table. If the number of studies is too large for this to be practical, this can be consigned to an appendix, or perhaps a "demographic summary" of the studies can be presented, much as one would describe age in a group of individuals as the mean age and the standard deviation. In some contexts, this layout is called an "evidence table." It should include all factors relevant to the qualitative assessment of the studies, without quantitative results. An example of such a table is Table 12-1.

Now we come to what is, arguably, the most critical yet difficult judgment to make: the combinability of the studies. The fundamental question is whether there exists a whole that is greater than the individual parts. It is important to make the rationale for this judgment explicit (although that is rarely done), and to base it partly without reference to the quantitative results. The only rational foundation for this judgment must be the proposed mechanism by which the intervention is thought to affect the outcome, and the possible modifiers of that effect. The question that the meta-analyst must be able to answer affirmatively is "In assessing the evidence for the efficacy of this intervention, is there more information in all of the studies considered together than there is in one study?" or, to make it more personal, "If I were making a decision about this relationship for myself, would I be interested only in the one study whose subjects or interventions matched my situation best, or would I want to see the results from other studies?" Often, considering these kinds of questions can reveal opinions about the underlying conceptual framework that are not clearly recognized when abstractly considering study methodology.

In the EFM example, components of this conceptual framework include the following:

- Processes that result in bad neonatal outcomes affect the fetus in ways that can often can be detected in their early stages through EFM (e.g., hypoxia with subsequent fetal heart rate change).
- That intervention on the basis of EFM can modify the process so as to reduce the chance of a bad outcome.
- That the effect of intervention on the basis of EFM is not highly dependent on patient medical or demographic characteristics, variations in the medical setting, or the exact intervention.
- That the effect of intervention on the basis of EFM is not highly dependent on the sensitivity of the procedure, which can be affected by monitoring criteria or personnel used to define fetal distress, or the use of fetal scalp sampling.

It is important to recognize that study eligibility criteria implicitly include judgments about permissible variability, and serve to reduce variability among the studies that are examined in depth. The justifications above are made only within the context of the studies that are candidates for pooling. There is often a tendency to make some of the above judgments solely on the basis of the quantitative results, but it is critical to make a qualitative judgment about them first. Two studies in completely different fields can have a RR = 2, but this does not mean they should be combined.

In the end, the judgment that any studies are combinable can always be challenged. The goal of both the process and reporting of a meta-analysis should be to present the argument for (or against) pooling in a manner that subsequent discussions of this issue can clearly be about the scientific issues that went into the judgment, rather than being unfocused rejections of the whole procedure based on its results.

Summary of Issues in Qualitative Assessment

1. All aspects of design features of studies that are relevant to the interpretation of their results should be included and presented in a large table.
2. Any relevant patterns or important differences in the designs of the studies should be noted in the text.
3. The reasons why various design features are relevant, or could have an impact on an individual study's result, should be stated in the text. This must be based on a clearly articulated mechanistic or conceptual framework.
4. The judgment that the studies should or should not be combined should be stated and justified explicitly.

Table 12-1. Qualitative factors relevant to studies relating colon cancer to fiber intake, with data

		Description of Study Populations			
Study Center	Location	Source of Cases and Years of Sampling	Control Source	Type of Matching	Matching Variables
Argentina	LaPlata	10 hospitals (1985–1987)	Neighborhood	Individual	Age, sex, residence
Australia	Adelaide	Cancer registry (1979–1980)	Electoral rolls	Individual	Age, sex
Belgium	Liege	Hospitals, clinics, laboratories (1978–1983)	Population registry	Frequency	Age, sex, province

Source: Friedenreich et al. (1994).

Quality Scoring

A quasi-quantitative way of describing the literature, while also assessing the studies' relative credibility, is to assign them scores relating to their "quality." The issue of assessing and incorporating study quality measurements into a meta-analysis is controversial. It is important because if the studies that go into a meta-analysis are of poor quality, either they may be systematically biased or the "weight" one accords to the findings should be less than the total numbers might indicate. Adding together biased studies not only will produce a biased result but will create an illusion of high precision. One solution to this is to rate the quality of the component studies and to use this quality score as either a weighting or exclusion (weight = 0) criterion. The problem is that there are a multitude of quality scoring indexes (Moher et al., 1995) but little agreement as to which of these is preferable or, indeed, if some composite quality score should ever be used (Detsky et al., 1992; Greenland, 1994). Strong arguments have been made that the components of a quality index, rather than the summary index, should be used as the basis for sensitivity analyses or as inputs into metaregression (to be discussed later). Perhaps the best way to view a quality score is as a descriptive tool to help collapse many qualitative dimensions. Whether these scores hide more than they show and whether the assessment of the reporting quality is a valid index of the research quality are questions that have to be answered for the specific set of studies being examined.

Because there are so many quality indexes (with few having been developed from the first three of the 13 studies that were examined

Dietary Assessment Methods					
Measurement Instrument	*Method of Administration*	*Time Period for Diet Reporting*	*Portion Size Estimated*	*Method for Portion Size*	*Frequency Measurement*
Food frequency	Interview	5-year period up to 6 months before interview	No	Standard portions from 1982 pilot study in Rosario, Argentina	6 categories
Food frequency	Self-interview	1 year before	Yes	Standard serving sizes	7 categories
Diet history organized by meals	Self-interview	1 year before disease onset	Yes	Photographs of standard portions	Absolute

for observational studies), many authors compose their own (e.g., Longnecker et al., 1988), borrowing from previous work and tailoring some questions specifically to the subject they are investigating. This is essentially what the authors of the electronic fetal monitoring meta-analysis did with the following list of quality criteria:

1. Prior hypotheses
2. Power calculation
3. Eligibility criteria
4. Randomization (random numbers, random weeks, alternate months, coin toss)
5. Withdrawals
6. Description of regimen
7. Adherence to regimen
8. Blinding of physicians
9. Blinding of statisticians
10. Unambiguous end points
11. Appropriate statistics for main effects
12. Appropriate statistics for subgroups
13. Complications of monitoring

Most of these are fairly generic randomized clinical trial assessment criteria, as contrasted with subject-specific scores that are occasionally constructed. Each of the above criteria was rated as "yes," "some," "no," or "unclear." The results of these ratings were presented as the first table of the paper. As can be seen from this list, it includes a combination of factors relating to reporting, study design, execution, and analysis. Separating the quality of the report from the quality of the study itself is not done well by any current quality assessment system, though the importance of that distinction is debated. In addition, often one or two critical factors may have overriding importance in a particular area. A good source for potential components of a quality index is the elements chosen for data abstraction. For example, in health services research, where training, compliance, and follow-up can be critical elements, the rigor with which each of these is assessed could be made part of a custom-made quality index. Whether a study is admitted for consideration and then down-weighted because of some serious flaw or instead excluded initially is an issue for the investigator to decide.

The exact method by which the authors of the electronic fetal monitoring meta-analysis constructed a summary quality index was not clear. They stated, "A score was given to each criterion, and the sum of the points assessed for each criterion was then divided by the total . . . possible . . . and converted to a percentage" (Thacker et al., 1995). We are not told how many points were assigned to each criterion or how much to intermediate scores. The results of this procedure were reported in summary form in the text, with the scores ranging from 29% to 86%. It should be clear that such composite summary scores allow only rather crude stratifications of studies since it is not always clear that the absence of some criterion (e.g., power calculations) necessarily has a material relation to the weight of the evidence a study provides. Some of these criteria are perhaps better viewed as surrogates; if a study is reported with a complete power calculation, it may be that other aspects of the quantitative analysis were done better than in studies that do not have one. However, the variation of study results with each of these components can be examined empirically in the quantitative component of the meta-analysis.

The following statements summarize the issues in quality assessment:

1. There are no widely accepted or validated quality assessment instruments for scientific studies, though many have been proposed, mainly for clinical trials.
2. Quality assessment is sometimes handled implicitly in the construction of eligibility criteria.
3. A quality scoring system can borrow from existing indexes but usually needs some specific tailoring to the subject at hand.
4. How the summary score was produced should be clear in the write-up of the meta-analysis.
5. The preferability of summary quality scores vs. using components of the

score in sensitivity analyses, stratified analyses, or metaregressions is an area of controversy.

6. Quality scores are useful only to make fairly crude distinctions between studies. The use of the specific score to produce a "weight" does not have validity.

Quantitative Data Abstraction

Finally, we come to the part of the meta-analytic procedure that many often think is its only component—the abstraction and pooling of results. The first question is what results need to be abstracted. If data are to be abstracted only from the published literature, this decision may have already been made by how other authors have reported their results. However, good meta-analyses often have obtained from authors data or results that did not appear in their reports, as the electronic fetal monitoring authors did:

> All corresponding authors were contacted for data not available in published reports, and all provided the requested information, when available (Thacker et al., 1995).

This is not always a luxury. Sometimes getting more data from the original investigators is a necessity. However, it is not always possible. Sometimes the investigators have moved, the data are no longer available, or the authors are simply unwilling to provide the requested results. However, the effort should always be made when the published data are incomplete or would lead to the exclusion of a study that could materially affect the conclusions or the precision of estimates.

The data to be abstracted usually include all important outcomes and potential confounders for each study in the meta-analysis, just as an individual clinical trial would record such details on each subject. The authors presented a large table with the following abstracted results:

1. Number of women
2. Number of infants
3. Maternal risk status
4. Fetal scalp blood sampling
5. Total of cesarean deliveries
6. Cesarean deliveries with fetal indications
7. Operative vaginal deliveries
8. 1 min apgar <7
9. 1 min apgar <4
10. Neonatal seizures
11. Admissions to neonatal intensive care units

12. Mean length of stay
13. Perinatal death rate
14. Stillbirths
15. Neonatal deaths

Data that were unpublished but provided by the authors were indicated in the tables, as were data that could not be verified by an author or were not available. If the number of studies is not excessive, it is critical that such a table be provided either in the body of a meta-analysis or as an appendix when it is published. This is the only way that other researchers can have access to the data being synthesized. Even if it is not published in its entirety, such a table must be compiled for the quantitative meta-analysis to be conducted.

For many outcomes, data may not be presented in exactly the form desired. For example, age might be reported as "% over 35" in one study, median age in another, and mean age in another. The meta-analyst must make decisions on how to handle this. Often, approximate data can be abstracted from figures and error bars or inferred from significance tests or from other data supplied in the text. The job of the meta-analyst is to decide what quantitative outcome measure strikes the right balance between maximum inclusivity and the elimination of so much that later pooling becomes meaningless.

Quantitative Meta-analysis

The complexity of meta-analytic statistical methodologies is growing rapidly (Cooper and Hedges, 1994), and it is beyond the scope of this presentation to review them all. Instead, we focus on the two simplest and most widely used methodologies to "add up" studies. The two sections on statistical methods are more technical than the preceding ones, so the reader not interested in equations may wish to skip those.

The first step in a quantitative meta-analysis mirrors those in the qualitative part: exploratory data analysis. The effect measures from each study (e.g., risk difference, odds ratios) should be displayed on a graph with their confidence intervals lined up so that the variation in study estimates can be clearly examined. An addition to the graphic element is making the size of the symbol at the effect estimate proportional to the sample size of that study because otherwise the smallest trials with the largest confidence intervals will attract the most attention. This display was pioneered by Richard Peto and is shown in Figure 12-1 (without the variable symbol size), which is taken from the meta-analysis on stroke units that we will examine later (Langhorne et al., 1993). This display can be ordered or stratified by various important trial characteristics (as it is here) to show any correlations between study characteristics and outcomes.

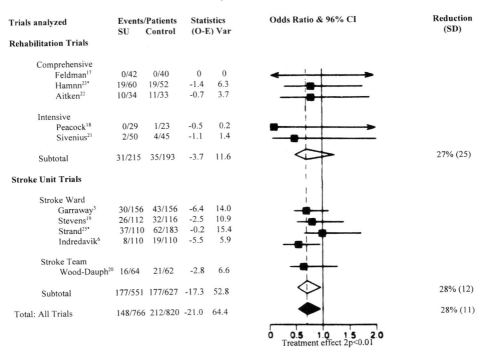

Figure 12-1. Short-term mortality results in the study of stroke units reported by Lang-horne et al. (1993). The trials are organized by design. Initial mortality after stroke: stroke unit (SU) vs. general wards (control). O-E indicates observed minus expected number of events in treatment (SU) group: var denotes variance. ■ = odds ratio of death in stroke unit group vs. in general wards for each trial with its 95% CI (horizontal line): ◇ = overview of trial results and 95%. CI: ◆ = total for all trials. Reduction = reduction in overall mortality for these trials. Broken vertical line is odds ratio for all available trials.

The choice of effect measure is a judgment with important implications. If there is no clear continuous metric (like blood pressure), the analyst has a variety of choices: for count data, an odds ratio, risk ratio, or risk difference; for continuous data, either an "effect size" defined relative to the population standard deviation or a discrete outcome based on categorizing the continuous measure (e.g., quality of life score as "low," "medium," or "high"). The only measure that should be avoided, if possible, is the standard deviation effect size since this often does not have biologic meaning and there is no necessary reason to imagine that it should be constant. However, particularly in psychometric or social research, where the instruments used to measure outcomes can vary widely, sometimes this statistical measure is the only choice. The fundamental principle behind the choice of an outcome measure is that it should be roughly constant across studies and consistent with the purposes of the meta-analysis. For example, multiplicative measures are often most appropriate for etiologic/causal questions, where absolute changes and risk differences are typically what is needed by policymakers and decision analysts. The constancy of these various measures should be examined empirically with the data in hand.

One factor that can be examined in this exploratory stage is the possibility of publication bias, that is, the tendency of either authors or journal editors (usually the former) not to publish statistically nonsignificant results. This can be examined informally (though there are statistical procedures to formally assess it, which we will not look at here). The most useful graphic tool to evaluate this is called a "funnel plot" (Fig. 12-2) (Light and Pillemer, 1984). The funnel plot is a graph of the point estimates of studies (x-axis) plotted against the standard error of each point estimate (y-axis). It is called a funnel plot because, in the absence of any publication bias, it should have roughly a funnel shape since, as the standard error increases, we would expect to see a spread of observed effects that extends over a larger range (approximately two standard errors in each direction). The cardinal sign of publication bias is a "hole" in the middle or on one side of the plot, that is, an area where we would expect to see study results but where there are apparently none. If the hole is in the middle, then we may suspect that trials with the most extreme results are being published, without the moderate (and

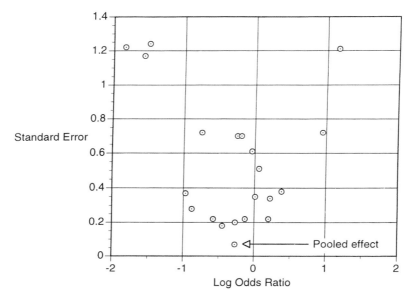

Figure 12-2. An example of a funnel plot. There appears to be a gap in the upper center of the plot, suggesting that small trials were published only if they showed rather extreme results. However, there is no evidence in this plot that this omission would systematically have biased the results, which would be likely only if one side of the plot were missing.

probably nonsignificant) ones in the middle. If one side of the plot seems to be missing trials, then it could be that effects in the direction opposite to the conventional opinion tend not to be published or that the most "positive" outcome measure is reported as the primary one. Formal statistical procedures to assess publication bias have been developed (Begg and Berlin, 1988; Dear and Begg, 1992; Hedges, 1992).

In the meta-analysis we are discussing, an effect measure of relative risk was used. This was applied to measure the effect on virtually all outcomes. Unfortunately, whereas raw data from the individual studies were presented in a large table, the summary effect measures were not presented by individual trial; only their sum was presented.

Statistical methods: fixed effects model

If the preceding steps have been done well, the quantitative meta-analysis should follow naturally and, at least from a technical perspective, should not have to be difficult. There are two basic approaches to quantitative meta-analysis. The first is a "weighted-sum" approach, where studies are assigned weights, usually based on the precision of the outcome measure being pooled, and the pooled estimate is the weighted sum of outcome measures. Confounders are controlled for in this approach by stratification, that is, calculating weighted averages within various strata of the possible confounders. The other general approach is a meta-regression model, wherein the possible confounders are entered as independent variables in a weighted regression, with the outcome measures as the dependent variables.

By far, the most common method has been the weighted average approach, so we will focus on that here. The basic equations for calculating the meta-analytic estimate of effect $\bar{m}$ (n = number of studies), are the following:

$$\bar{m} = \frac{\sum_i^n w_i m_i}{\sum_i^n w_i}$$

where w_i is weight and m_1 is any normally distributed outcome measure, which can include both continuous variables or, for dichotomous outcomes, the log odds ratio [In (OR_1)] or risk difference ($RD_1 = p_{i1} - p_{i2}$).

$$\text{weight} = w_i = \frac{1}{\text{variance } (m_i)}$$

$$\text{Variance } [\ln (OR_i)] = \frac{1}{a_i} + \frac{1}{b_i} + \frac{1}{c_i} + \frac{1}{d_i}$$

$$\text{Variance } (RD_i) = \frac{p_{i1}q_{i1}}{n_{i1}} + \frac{p_{i2}q_{i2}}{n_{i2}}$$

The variance of this meta-analytic average is the reciprocal of the sum of the weights:

$$\text{variance } (\bar{m}) = \frac{1}{\displaystyle\sum_{i=1}^{n} \text{weight}_i}$$

What these equations say is that the result of each study is assigned a weight proportional to its precision (defined as 1/variance): the higher the precision (corresponding to a smaller variance), the higher the weight. Since larger sample sizes typically produce more precise estimates, larger studies typically get higher weight, which is what we would expect.

When the information being synthesized comes in the form of proportions that can be expressed in 2 × 2 tables, the best formula for synthesis is the standard Mantel-Haenszel formula for combining odds ratios from separate strata:

$$\text{Mantel-Haenszel OR} = \sum_{i=1}^{n} \frac{a_i d_i / n_i}{b_i c_i / n_i}$$

Where i is study number; n_i is sample size of the ith study; n is number of studies; and a_i, b_i, c_i, and d_i are the entries in the ith study's 2 × 2 table.

There is an assumption, however, built into all of these formulas that needs to be checked before using them. What these formulas implicitly say is that all of the observed difference between the studies is due to chance. That is, each of the studies is attempting to estimate the same true effect, and the only reason the study results differ is statistical fluctuation. It is only under this assumption that combining studies in this way is justified. The technical name for this way of thinking about the sources of variation among studies is the "fixed effects model." If, in fact, certain studies had patients, interventions, or some other characteristic that meant the effect measured in that study should be different, it would not make sense to combine it with others to estimate a "typical" effect, which may apply to none of the studies. Therefore, we must check this assumption statistically before we apply this formula. This check is called a "test of homogeneity," that is, a test that the observed scatter of study outcomes is consistent with all of them estimating the same underlying effect. The formula for the test of homogeneity is the following:

$$Q = \chi^2_{\text{homo}} = \sum_{i=1}^{n} w_i(m_i - \bar{m})^2$$

where degrees of freedom are $n - 1$.

Briefly, the test takes the difference between each study's effect and the fixed-effects pooled estimate, squares it, multiplies it by that study's weight, and adds them up across all of the studies. This is distributed approximately as a chi-squared statistic with $n - 1$ degrees of freedom.

This test must be applied to studies being meta-analyzed before any other quantitative manipulations. One of the problems, however, is that the test has relatively low power when there are few studies (e.g., Light and Pillemer, 1984; Longnecker et al., 1988; Detsky et al., 1992; Greenland, 1994). This means that there can be a fairly high variability among studies but that p value may be above the usual significance threshold of 0.05. Therefore, a threshold p value of 0.10–0.15 is typically used when there are few studies.

It is often said that if there is statistical heterogeneity, the meta-analysis should not proceed. However, there are several options at this point. First and foremost, the studies must be examined closely to see if the reason for their wide variation in effect can be explained by the differences among study designs, populations, etc. If this is found, the analysis can be stratified by that factor and subgroups of studies that are homogeneous on that factor can be combined. Alternatively, one can turn to a ''random effects'' model, which we present next.

Statistical methods: random effects model

Another model used to synthesize evidence in meta-analyses is called the ''random effects model'' (DerSimonian and Laird, 1986). This model is particularly useful in the face of apparent heterogeneity, though, as we will see below, it is not necessarily appropriate when the heterogeneity is extreme. The underlying assumption of this model is that the true effect underlying each study is different; therefore, they are not all estimating the same effect. In other words, the studies are somewhat heterogeneous. The model assumes that studies differ because of all of the aspects that can affect outcome: different populations, different treatments, different follow-up, different methods of outcome ascertainment, etc. However, while it is acknowledged that studies differ, it is still assumed that there is a meaningful common effect from which each study differs but that the degree of difference from that common effect is not so great as to make the purported common effect meaningless.

This issue can be illustrated with a simple example. Suppose we have three studies that report odds ratios of 2, 3, and 5. It could be reasonable in this situation to postulate that some of this variation is due to statistical fluctuation and some to the difference between studies but that some "average" odds ratio near 3 or 4 could still represent an approximate summary of the effect of the intervention, so a random effects model would make sense. If, however, the odds ratios are more dramatically different—for example, 0.2, 0.8, and 5—there really cannot be a "typical" odds ratio. The average of around 3 is observed in none of the studies, and it is unclear whether the intervention is harmful or beneficial. In a situation like this, the "common" odds ratio, even if derived with a random effects model, is not a fair representation of the typical effect. So a reasonable choice would be to not formally combine these results at all, at least until the wide disparity in effect sizes can be explained. This is an area of judgment in meta-analyses that is sometimes difficult, and it is best to work with an experienced biostatistician if problems of heterogeneity arise.

To return to the mathematics, the basic equations of the random effects model are not difficult, though the principles underlying the method are a bit tricky. We start by presenting the two stages of the model: the variation of each study's true mean around the common effect and the variation (due to statistical fluctuation) of each study's observed mean around its true mean. This is written below in the two-stage model of the random effects formulas.

First stage:

$$q_i = U + d_i$$

where q_i is the true effect that the ith trial is trying to estimate; U is the "grand mean" overall effect, averaged over all trial types and study populations; and d_i is the deviation due to differences in study population, design, or other study-specific factors.

Second stage:

$$m_i = \theta_i + e_i$$

where m_i is the observed effect in the ith trial; θ_i is the true effect that the ith trial is trying to estimate; and e_i is the deviation due to pure statistical error, that is, not to differences in study population or design. The e_i values have variance of σ_i^2, calculated as in the fixed-effects model. The d_i values have variance of τ^2, which can be estimated as follows:

$$\hat{\tau}^2 = \frac{Q - (n - 1)}{\left(\sum_{i=1}^{n} w_i - \dfrac{\sum_{i=1}^{n} w_i^2}{\sum_{i=1}^{n} w_i} \right)}$$

where Q is the fixed effects test of homogeneity.

We now recalculate the variance of each trial observation as the sum of the sampling variance (σ_i^2) and the variance due to study factors (τ^2). This allows us to recalculate the study weights and then to use the fixed effects formula for a weighted average:

$$\overset{\frown}{\text{variance}} * (m_i) = \hat{\sigma}_i^2 + \hat{\tau}^2 = \text{random effects variance for study } i$$

$$\text{weight} * (m_i) = 1/\overset{\frown}{\text{variance}} * (m_i) = \text{random effects weight for study } i$$

There are a variety of other methods currently being used to handle the problem of heterogeneity, most notably metaregression, where various study characteristics are put in a regression equation to adjust the common estimate for study differences (Greenland, 1994). These are not yet widely used, and they will not be presented here. However, because of the heterogeneity that is more often seen in observational studies than in randomized clinical trials, these tools can be expected to be quite useful in exploring the reasons behind differences in studies of health services interventions.

Quantitative meta-analysis: example

We will now see how many of the preceding issues were dealt with in the example being studied in this chapter.

> Before combining risk estimates from multiple RCTs, we determined whether the study design and implementation were comparable. We did not combine data from studies that did not specifically address the comparative efficacy of continuous EFM and auscultation; results from these trials are presented separately. (Thacker et al., 1995)

The authors have prospectively stated aspects of study design that they feel define a homogeneous group of interventions and outcomes. It is good to establish this before the results are seen because the near-equality of effect sizes is not sufficient justification for combining; the study designs and outcomes have to be similar enough so that the synthesis is meaningful and interpretable.

> Because of the small number of neonatal seizures, we pooled these data from the original studies rather than pooling risk estimates. For the remaining outcomes, we weighted each study's risk estimate by its inverse variance and computed an overall estimate as the weighted average. (Thacker et al., 1995)

Most of the formulas presented earlier do not work well with very small numbers. In those situations, we must use either more sophisticated methods or the option these investigators used, that is, the original data, not the summary estimates of effect.

> We tested for heterogeneity by using the method of DerSimonian and Laird. If significant heterogeneity was present ($p < 0.10$), we reported estimates from the random effects model. (Thacker et al., 1995)

The authors use a slightly more liberal definition of statistical heterogeneity than $p < 0.05$, which is good. In those situations, they use the random effects model. However, as mentioned previously, excessive or qualitative heterogeneity is not automatically taken care of adequately by the random effects model; the option to not combine studies at all must always be open.

> Cumulative calculations assessing the total estimated effect as further studies were complete were done for five of the outcomes. . . . In addition, we performed cumulative meta-analyses according to increasing quality score and increasing study size. (Thacker et al., 1995)

This is a very useful exploratory and display technique: to order the studies according to some measure (the most common of which is time) and to present an accumulating sum of the studies as a function of that measure.

The results of the meta-analysis are presented by these authors in tables, figures, and text. In brief, the results were as follows. Morbidity end points included 1 min Apgar score and seizures. Only seven studies reported percentages of newborns with Apgar scores less than 4, and in these, monitoring showed a slight protective effect (relative risk [RR] = 0.82, 95% confidence interval [CI] 0.65–0.98), which the authors noted was due to non-U.S. studies. They reported RR = 0.50 for neonatal seizures, 95% CI 0.30–0.82, an effect they said was evident only in the "high quality" studies. They reported no overall effect on perinatal death (RR = 0.76, 95% CI 0.04–1.39), with a p value for heterogeneity of 0.04, but noted a strong effect in non-U.S. studies (RR = 0.21, 95% CI 0.12–0.29). Finally, they reported an elevation in the number of operative deliveries, both vaginal and cesarean, RR = 1.23, 95% CI 1.15–1.31. Interestingly, the authors do not report p values for any end point.

How are we to interpret such findings? We will examine this in our look at the authors' discussion section, but a few points are worth making now. First, since a meta-analysis is an observational study, the weight we might want to put on a "just significant" result may be less than the weight we would apply to the same result from a randomized clinical trial or well-done prospective study. In other words, results with p values in at least the 0.01–0.05 range should probably be regarded as somewhat tentative (Goodman, 1989). These would correspond to confidence intervals that came fairly close to the null effect.

Second, the manner in which subgroup effects were analyzed and reported here is problematic. As in a clinical trial, the proper analysis for the existence of a subgroup effect would be to test whether the effect in that subgroup statistically differed from the effect measured in the remaining subjects. This is akin to a test for heterogeneity. Noting a significant effect in one subgroup and a nonsignificant one in the remainder does not mean that results in the two groups are inconsistent and that a subgroup effect can be claimed. Examining the overlap in the CIs between the subgroups is a good clue as to whether there is statistical evidence for a subgroup effect: no overlap means there is a fair amount of statistical evidence, small overlap is equivocal, and wide overlap (which is usually the case) means the results are statistically compatible.

These authors presented their meta-analysis of 12 trials with the following sequence of tables and figures:

Table 1: the rating of each of the quality components of every trial
Table 2: quantitative results of nine outcome measures, with a footnoted design description of each trial
Table 3: summary odds ratio, 95% CI, and heterogeneity tests for five main end points
Table 4: cumulative (by date) summary odds ratio for five main end points
Table 5: summary odds ratio, 95% CI, and heterogeneity tests for three safety-related end points
Figure: cumulative meta-analytic summary of risk of neonatal seizures

This is an interesting and fairly good model of the sequence and nature of data that should be presented in a meta-analysis. The parallel cumulative meta-analyses of multiple end points is a particularly interesting and unusual touch, though a figure would have been a better medium to convey that information. One striking omission, however, is the absence of any displays of the effect estimates of individual trials, as in our Figure 12-1. Although the data are reported in their Table 2, a visual image of the individual trial data is an extraordinarily useful way to communicate complex patterns involving multiple end points. Although the narrative summary in the text is quite complete, we nevertheless are not left with as good a sense of the variability between studies as a picture can convey.

Another problem in this meta-analysis is its exclusive use of multiplicative measures of relative effect. This precludes appropriate risk–benefit comparison. For example, the relative risk for the reduction of neonatal seizures was 0.50, whereas that for the increase in operative deliveries was 1.23. To make a rational assessment of the trade-off, we need to know the baseline risks, which would allow us to measure the absolute increase or decrease in both event rates. Close examination of the tabular data shows that the number of operative deliveries was approximately 15 times more than the number of neonatal seizures. Thus, a 25% increase in the number of those deliveries represents about eight times more additional operative deliveries than neonatal seizures prevented by halving the seizure rate. Whether this was an appropriate balance may be beyond the scope of a meta-analysis to determine, but the numbers should always be presented in such a way that this contrast can be made.

The one aspect of quantitative meta-analysis that has not been mentioned is a sensitivity analysis. This involves exploring the sensitivity of the results to the exclusion of either single trials, groups of trials, or any of the methodologic assumptions employed in the analysis. This is increasingly recognized as a critical component of all meta-analyses. For some meta-analysts, finding the possible determinants or correlates of effect size, which can be viewed as "explaining heterogeneity," is a primary goal of what others might call a sensitivity analysis (e.g., Pladevall-Vila et al., 1996). This perspective transforms a finding of heterogeneity in effect size from an obstacle to be overcome to a natural phenomenon that should be studied. In the electronic fetal monitoring meta-analysis, the text reports the results of various exclusions of studies for various end points, which constitutes a de facto sensitivity analysis.

The following statements summarize the issues in quantitative meta-analysis:

1. The initial step of quantitative synthesis should be a quantitative exploration and display of the data both to effectively communicate individual trial data and to explore the implications of using different outcome measures (e.g., odds ratio vs. risk difference).
2. The next step is an analysis of heterogeneity, based both on the study design characteristics and on the quantitative outcomes. Quantitative synthesis must proceed in the face of heterogeneity with great caution and expert technical assistance.
3. Individual trial results of main outcomes should be presented, if possible, as figures and tables.
4. The primary statistical method must be selected, with the main choice being between fixed effects and random effects summaries. Methods to handle confounding or heterogeneity include stratified analyses and meta-regression.
5. Sensitivity analysis should be performed on all design and clinical characteristics potentially relevant to the outcome.
6. The weight put on the resulting p value should be less than what would apply to the same p value in a single study of the same size as the meta-analysis and of the same design as the component studies used in the meta-analysis. In other words, an informal threshold for claiming the significance of $p < 0.01$ or $p < 0.001$ should be used.

Limitations, Conclusions, and Implications

One of the most persistent criticisms of meta-analysis is that its quantitative conclusions are accorded too much weight, either because the studies being combined are uncombinable or because the process of combination obscures the poor quality of underlying components (Shapiro, 1994; Spitzer, 1995). Most of the guidelines outlined in this chapter are aimed at addressing those criticisms,

ensuring that the studies being meta-analyzed are understood well enough understood for their combination to be reasonable and that their failings are understood
well enough so that their combination gets appropriate weight. However, the
bases for these judgments can get lost in the welter of statistics that typify the
results section of meta-analyses, and it is incumbent on authors to present in
the discussion section a clear, qualitative picture of the limitations of their
analysis. The best antidote for this problem is a sophisticated discussion of the
mechanism by which a proposed intervention should work, supported by empirical data and integrated with the quantitative results.

Another critical component of the discussion section is an examination of the
policy context in which the analysis occurs and of the anticipated effect of the
meta-analysis. Meta-analysis is somewhat unique insofar as it presents in summary form research that usually has been published already, and the motivation to
perform a meta-analysis is often explicitly to affect policy at some level. Policymakers presumably have had prior access to all of the relevant research, and in a
perfect world, health policy should already reflect it. If that is not true (generally
the rule), it can be extremely illuminating for the meta-analyst to examine why
current policy is seemingly at variance with the published research. This will
clearly help position the meta-analysis in terms of its hoped-for impact. If it is
simply the case that individual studies were too small to demonstrate differences
that would be important in populations, then the meta-analysis has essentially
produced a "new" result and the response to the individual trials may not be
predictive of the response to the meta-analysis. However, if the meta-analysis
merely strengthens conclusions that several large studies had already drawn, the
situation may be more complex. It is not the meta-analyst's job to provide a
political analysis of the current policy, but the issues that possibly have impeded
movement before should be clearly articulated so that it is clear why and in what
way the meta-analysis might help to inform policy where the individual studies
could not.

Of course, the results of a meta-analysis may not be definitive or provide a
clear direction for policy. This can be an important contribution in itself, showing
that current policy is not definitively supported by research evidence of effectiveness and pointing the way to future research.

Thacker et al. (1995) provide an excellent summary of the policy context of
their meta-analysis. They point out that 74% of pregnancies were monitored
electronically in the United States in 1992 but that both official bodies and expert
panels in the late 1980s had become skeptical enough so that electronic fetal
monitoring was not endorsed by these bodies for use in either low- or high-risk
pregnancies. They note that some of the randomized clinical trials they examined
were responsible for this change in attitude and that the initial introduction of fetal
monitoring occurred before any such trials had been conducted. They note that

this is yet another example of a technology that became widespread before its efficacy and safety were determined, leading to "misuse, misunderstanding, and unnecessary concerns regarding malpractice and litigation" (Thacker et al., 1995).

They summarize their findings, distinguishing between strong and weak results. They state that, with the exception of a reduction in the rate of neonatal seizures, routine electronic fetal monitoring had no measurable impact on the morbidity or mortality of infants. They note that the long-term effects of the seizures are probably minimal and that the evidence for some subgroup findings must be regarded as preliminary. They note that the most striking and consistent adverse outcome was a rise in the number of operative deliveries. Their final summary tells us where they see these results fitting into current policy and the future research direction:

> What do the RCTs tell us about the appropriate use of the EFM in clinical practice? The benefits once claimed for the EFM are clearly more modest than once believed, and appear to be primarily in the prevention of neonatal seizures. However, the long-term implications of this outcome appear less serious than once believed. . . . At the same time, the risks associated with the use of EFM, especially the risk of caesarean delivery, appear to have been reduced but not eliminated. [NB: This is where a quantitative contrast of the two risks would have been very useful.]
>
> Much remains to be learned about the intrapartum period and its long-term effects on the fetus. Future RCTs in this arena should focus on clearly specified clinical questions: 1) Which groups might benefit most from intrapartum surveillance? 2) What are the essential or desirable elements of this technique? and 3) What is the long-term follow-up of children in the 12 studies already conducted? (Thacker et al., 1995)

The following statements summarize the issues in discussion/conclusions.

1. The limitations of the meta-analysis must be clearly outlined so that it is clear what weight the authors feel should be put on the verdict.
2. The policy background should be clear so that it is obvious in what way this meta-analysis should affect policy in any way different from prior published research.
3. The interpretation of results needs to be clearly linked to a discussion of the proposed mechanism by which the intervention has its positive or adverse effect.
4. The meta-analysis, by pointing out weaknesses in the empirical evidence base, should show where future research can be improved or directed. Authors should also comment on whether more research is, in fact, needed; sometimes an outcome is so definitive that the ethics of continued research can be questioned.

Stroke Unit Example

A meta-analysis by Langhorne et al. (1993) on the effect of specialized stroke units in the morbidity and mortality resulting from stroke illustrates some of the practical difficulties that can be encountered when applying the technique of meta-analysis within health services research. We will not review this study in the same depth as the previous example but, instead, will highlight some of the problems these investigators encountered, which are likely to be seen in other health services meta-analyses.

They state that their primary outcome was mortality within 17 weeks of stroke, though causes of death were usually not available and functional outcomes were measured in too many different ways to be combinable. Their mortality results are shown in Figure 12-1. The trials found were conducted over a very long time interval: one as early as 1962 and the last in 1993. The reader might wonder if the difference in ancillary care across decades could have impacted on the effect observed within the trials.

Another problem confronted by these meta-analysts was that "specialized stroke units" was very broadly defined. Some were specialized stroke wards, one was a mobile stroke team, and the others were more intensive or comprehensive packages of stroke rehabilitation. This is a problem most likely to confront studies of health services intervention; health services interventions aimed at the same outcome can be widely disparate. If the meta-analyst wants to add up the results from such different interventions, an explicit rationale must be provided in the qualitative analysis section. Although the authors of this meta-analysis note many of the differences between the trials, they justify their combination by noting the "homogeneity of mortality results" and because "[a]ll trials involved a specialist multidisciplinary team that provided continuity of care during the first few weeks of illness" (Langhorne et al., 1993).

The latter reason constitutes a qualitative justification (albeit one that could be argued), whereas the former, quantitative reason does not; that kind of rationale could be used to combine studies of any medical treatments that produced a 30% mortality decrease. Just because two interventions have the same effect on an outcome does not mean that we are justified in claiming twice the evidence in support of both of them.

The authors of this meta-analysis note in their conclusions that, because of the heterogeneity of the details of the interventions, their overview "does not indicate which interventions improve survival" (Langhorne et al., 1993). Their final conclusion was that there was "sufficient evidence to recommend better organized specialist stroke services that would, in turn, facilitate studies of specific components of stroke unit practice" (Langhorne et al., 1993).

This meta-analysis is an excellent one to reflect on because it embodies many of the strengths and weaknesses of the application of this methodology in the health services arena. The strength is that the authors were able to give us a clear picture of the evidence base (in the form of randomized clinical trials) for this practice and the variety of interventions and outcomes that had been studied. They also showed that, while few of the individual studies demonstrated statistically significant decreases in mortality, almost all were in the direction of decreasing mortality and that looking at them together strongly suggested a beneficial effect. Whether they should have been quantitatively combined, however, remains a legitimate question. This problem is reflected in the authors' inability to identify what aspect, or even category, of stroke service is likely to be beneficial. It is hard to argue against their recommendation that these units be "better organized" and that further study be done, but whether there is enough empirical evidence, for example, to justify a national policy of instituting such specialist-staffed units (which they did not specifically advocate) remains an open question. This is an excellent example of how meta-analysis can help to clarify the relevant issues and, perhaps, restrict or target the areas of real controversy, but it may not always settle them. The consumer needs to know how to look behind the mathematics to the judgments that underlie decisions about what, when, and how to combine study results.

Conclusion

Meta-analysis is a potentially powerful new technique to systematically review, analyze, and synthesize the body of research on a specific health care intervention. It can focus on both strengths and weaknesses in the empirical evidence base that were previously overlooked, either because the evidence base was not reviewed systematically or because individual studies were too small to be able to accurately measure an intervention's impact. The challenge to the meta-analyst and to the consumers of these types of systematic review is to assess whether the research is consistent enough in design and purpose to justify combining results and, if combined, what weight to put on them. The proper use of this method can lead to a closer tie between health policy decisions and the evidence that supports the effectiveness and safety of those policies.

References

Begg, C., J. Berlin. 1988. Publication bias: a problem in interpreting medical data. *J. R. Stat. Soc. A.*, 151:419–463.

Bero, L., D. Rennie. 1995. The Cochrane Collaboration. Preparing, maintaining, and disseminating systematic reviews of the effects of health care. *JAMA*, 274:1935–1938.

Blair, A., J. Burg, J. Foran, et al. 1995. Guidelines for application of meta-analysis in environmental epidemiology. *Regul. Toxicol. Pharmacol.*, 22:189–197.

Cooper, H., L. Hedges. 1994. *Handbook of Research Synthesis.* New York: Russel Sage Foundation.

Dear K., and C. Begg. 1992. An approach for assessing publication bias prior to performing a meta-analysis. *Statistical Science*, 7:237–245.

DerSimonian R., and N. Laird. 1986. Meta-analysis in clinical trials. *Control. Clin. Trials*, 7:177–188.

Detsky, A., C. Naylor, K. O'Rourke, et al. 1992. Incorporating variations in the quality of individual randomized trials into meta-analysis. *J. Clin. Epidemiol.*, 45:255–265.

Dickersin K., P. Hewitt, L. Mutch, et al. 1985. Comparison of MEDLINE searching with a perinatal clinical trials database. *Control. Clin. Trials*, 6:306–317.

Dickersin K., K. Higgins, and C. Meinert. 1990. Identification of meta-analyses: the need for standard terminology. *Control. Clin. Trials*, 11:52–66.

Dickersin K., Y. Min, and C. Meinert. 1991. Factors influencing publication of research results: follow-up of applications submitted to two institutional review boards. *JAMA*, 267:374–378.

Friedenreich, C. 1993. Methods for pooled analyses of epidemiologic studies. *Epidemiology*, 4:295–302.

Friedenreich, C., R. Brant, E. Riboli. 1994. Influence of methodologic factors in a pooled anaylsis of 13 case-control studies of colorectal cancer and dietary fiber. *Epidemiology*, 5:66–79.

Glass, G. 1976. Primary, secondary and meta-analysis of research. *Educ. Res.*, 5:3–9.

Goodman, S. 1989. Meta-analysis and evidence. *Control. Clin. Trials*, 10:188–204, errata 435.

Greenland, S. 1994. A critical look at some popular meta-analytic methods. *Am. J. Epidemiol.*, 140:290–296.

Hedges, L. 1992. Modeling publication selection effects in meta-analysis. *Statistical Science*, 7:246–255.

Langhorne, P., B. O'Williams, W. Gilchrist, et al. 1993. Do stroke units save lives? *Lancet*, 342:395–398.

Light, R., and D. Pillemer. 1984. *Summing Up: The Science of Reviewing Research.* Cambridge, MA: Harvard University Press.

Longnecker, M., J. Berlin, M. Orza, et al. 1988. A meta-analysis of alcohol consumption in relation to risk of breast cancer. *JAMA*, 260:652–656.

Moher, D., A. Jadad, G. Nichol, et al. 1995. Assessing the quality of randomized controlled trials: an annotated bibliography of scales and checklists. *Control. Clin. Trials*, 16:62–73.

Pladevall-Vila, M., G. Delclos, C. Varas, et al. 1996. Controversy of oral contraceptives and risk of rheumatoid arthritis: meta-analysis of conflicting studies and review of conflicting meta-analyses with special emphasis on analysis of heterogeneity. *Am. J. Epidemiol.*, 144:1–14.

Shapiro, S. 1994. Meta-analysis/shmeta-analysis. *Am. J. Epidemiol.*, 140:771–778.

Spitzer, W. 1995. The challenge of meta-analysis. *J. Clin. Epidemiol.*, 48:1–4.

Thacker, S., D. Stroup, and H. Peterson. 1995. Efficacy and safety of intrapartum electronic fetal monitoring: an update. *Obstet. Gynecol.*, 86:613–620.

Index